The Moral Discourse of Health in Modern Cairo

The Moral Discourse of Health in Modern Cairo

Persons, Bodies, and Organs

Mohammed Tabishat

LEXINGTON BOOKS
Lanham • Boulder • New York • Toronto • Plymouth, UK

Published by Lexington Books
A wholly owned subsidiary of Rowman & Littlefield
4501 Forbes Boulevard, Suite 200, Lanham, Maryland 20706
www.rowman.com

10 Thornbury Road, Plymouth PL6 7PP, United Kingdom

British Library Cataloguing in Publication Information Available

Library of Congress Cataloging-in-Publication Data
Tabishat, Mohammed, 1963-
The moral discourse on health in modern Cairo : persons, bodies, and organs / Mohammed Tabishat.
pages cm
Includes bibliographical references and index.
ISBN 978-0-7391-7979-6 (cloth : alk. paper) — ISBN 978-0-7391-7980-2 (electronic)
1. Medical anthropology—Egypt—Cairo. 2. Medical care—Egypt—Cairo. 3. Public health—Egypt—Cairo. 4. Traditional medicine—Egypt—Cairo. 5. Cairo (Egypt)—Social life and customs. I. Title.
GN296.5.E3T23 2014
362.10962'16—dc23

2013048077

∞™ The paper used in this publication meets the minimum requirements of American National Standard for Information Sciences—Permanence of Paper for Printed Library Materials, ANSI/NISO Z39.48-1992.

Printed in the United States of America

To my mother and the memory of my father,
both of whom made everything possible for me.

To my four wonderful children,
Tamima, Tala, Talal, and Tuleen,
and my wife Safaa.

Contents

Figures

Tables

Acknowledgments

I feel grateful for all the people who gave me help to complete this book. First, my sincere thanks to Gilbert Lewis from the University of Cambridge for reading, commenting, and assisting in developing the argument of this study. Without Gilbert's initial constructive criticism, insightful suggestions, my study could have never developed in the way it did. My heart-felt thanks to Talal Asad who has always provided me with invaluable intellectual support and has been an indispensable source of inspiration. Unforgettable too is the moral and intellectual support I received from Marilyn Strathern and Keith Hart.

The original study that led to the development of this book was generously supported by The Cambridge Overseas Trust, represented by Karim Rida Said Scholarship and Gonville and Guise. During the field research in Cairo, I was supported by a generous grant from the Population Council. Earnest thanks go out to Dr. Seteney Shami for reading my initial research plans and meeting with me during the subsequent stages of fieldwork. I also appreciate the help and encouragement of the late Cynthia Nelson from the American University in Cairo and Shahnaz Rouse from Sarah Lawrence College for reading and commenting on my work.

My loving gratitude goes to my friends in Cambridge and New York City where I lived and studied for several years. First is my friend, or rather brother, Sanjay Reddy. Our continuing friendship has never been interrupted for the last two decades or more. Many special thanks to David Mitchell, Volker Scheid, and David Dickinson. Gloria Pungutti, Betania Araujo, Catarina Cazanova, Alonso Barros, Alex Moore, Bassam Ali, Agnieszka Halemba, Saad al-Omari, Richard Griftin, thank you for your invaluable support and friendship. Most special and everlasting sense of gratefulness for the generous help of my friend Khadidjah Mattar for editing parts of different versions of my work from the beginning right to the very end of submitting the manuscript. My friends, your ideas will have their stamp on this study and well beyond.

In New York City where I was an exchange student at the New School for Social Research, I was privileged to study and receive the advice of Rayna Rapp, Veena Das, and Kate Crehan among others. The motivation I felt at the New School was incomparable to any other place I attended. There too, I was blessed to be friends with Tanya Baker. I will always feel indebted to her absolutely invaluable and indescribable kindness and support. My friends Laura Rouch, Charles Hirschkind, Robin Le Baron, Paulette Spencer, Jon Wilson, Ali Alwan, Mohammad Dagman, Randa Hafez, and Raghda Hafez (may her soul rest in peace). Last but not least I wish to thank Petra Kuppinger who shared the fieldwork experience with me.

In Cairo, I met and have been helped by people who became and still are very special friends. I particularly thank Dr. Magdy Said for his support and friendship. For him, I will always be thankful for our friendship and inspiring conversations. Many others gave me help and encouragement: Said Samir, Tamir Mahamoud, Warda Mahmoud, Iman Mirsal, and Michael Freschkopf.

Last but certainly not the least are the families of *Būlāq* and all the persons who shared their experiences and feelings of pain and joy. I would never forget how much Shami, Um Sahar, Um Ashraf, Um Karim, Abu Hassan, Fatma, and of course Hag Sukkar helped. For those and the many others I send my deepest appreciation for their hospitality and sharing their sense of happiness and sorrow with me. To these people and to the whole city of Cairo (the safe town—*al-balad al-amīn*) I send my love.

Back home we say, "the end often goes for the dearest" (*al-tāli la al-ghawāli*). My love, respect, and appreciation go for my big family including my wife Safaa and daughters Tamima, Tala, and Tuleen, and son Talal. For everyone in my family I say that the sense of life and hope in your eyes helped me complete my work. Your love is totally indescribable. It is impossible to live without it. My whole love goes to my mother, sisters, and brothers. To all of them I say, sorry for being away this long, parts of me however have always been with you, despite the distance.

Introduction

Society in Medicine and Health Care

Health and disease, wellness and illness, healing and sickness, life and death, are all familiar. They are all human conditions. But what do they mean in different societies? How are they perceived? How are they related to each other? What are the means to treat them, both cognitively and practically? How is treatment organized? What does it mean? And who participates in it? What is the role of each? How are these roles related to each other? And, for example, are its meanings shared evenly among different genders, age groups, or social classes, for example? Most profoundly, are these confined to issues of health and illness alone? Or they are meaningful in other fields of life, such as the family, religion, the law, or politics?

This book is concerned with all these questions but focuses on the last one. The answer is, yes. The ideas and practices used in health care are ultimately about life as a whole. They are significant in all social spheres. The various ways they are defined, circulated, and redefined therefore reveal fundamental aspects of the different ways society is organized. Most profoundly, health and illness and the various therapies used to maintain and treat them are socially valuable. Their values relate to social relations in both direct and indirect ways. As such, they contribute to preserving and/or challenging the social order at large. This book is concerned with exploring how this process occurs. Based on an ethnographic study in Cairo it views the city's health care practices as plural—composed of elements rooted in different traditions[1] including most notably modern biochemical medicine and Islamic-Greek medicine. In addition, they include elements from homeopathy, traditional Chinese medicine, and ancient Egyptian medicine. Of course, health-related practices somehow follow a logic derived from the society's long-standing traditions, which themselves result from prolonged processes of interaction between different systems concerned with healing. This is why I view the existing health practices in Cairo as composite forms consisting of elements rooted in different traditions and ameliorated to respond to the health concerns uniquely characterizing life in the city and the country as a whole.

My argument is that health care practices in Egypt constitute an index to read the way political, economic, and social conditions are experienced by those who use, embody, or live them and cope with their outcomes. I suggest viewing them not as a purely technical means to overcome discrete ailments but rather as a slice of a far more complex social effort to sustain and promote life in general. I hold that these practices carry the code of the sociocultural matrix in which they are embedded; they speak of the rationalities of different help-seeking efforts. In doing so, they represent the moral principles underlying the social efforts to alleviate pain and maintain life as a whole. Health-related practices in this sense constitute a critical platform to feel and live in both the physical and moral sense. The fact that they are plural makes them suitable for examining the particular logic that drives the different ways the local population manage different resources. This book starts with health practitioners and laypersons engaged in continuous pursuit to maintain their wellness and alleviate various kinds of pain. Their practices indicate a major concern with the morality of the medical practice. I view morality as a trope summing up a specific cultural capacity called *al-nafs*, which means the soul or the person but extends to accommodate the living conditions of the entire society. It is the local cultural space where the subject and subjectivities are made and remade. It mirrors the relationship between individuals and society as it assists in both coping with and remaking the socioeconomic and political conditions through the force of emotions. These play a major role in expressing pain as well as in transforming physical categories of biomedicine into moral means to criticizing the dominant orders. The latter is perceived as unjust and therefore destructive to desired sense of wellness. Finally, perceptions are viewed not as static and monolithic but rather as continuously changing under the effect of debates that include the entire tradition they belong to.

AN ORIENTATION

I discuss the aforementioned questions in the context of field research in Cairo. I first explore the health resources available to the population. I further identify the way these are organized. Do they live in harmony? We all know that modern biomedicine is the major and more important medical system in the country. But how does it operate? When used how is it aligned to other kinds of therapy? People have long used different therapies simultaneously. What are the implications of this process of combining not only the therapies but the moral and social assumptions underlying them? In this study I include an underrepresented form of medical care, which is self-help. I examine a number of health pamphlets and focus on the different ways practitioners introduce their therapies in critical ways. I mean how they shift their relative physical and moral significance. My concern is to look into the sociopolitical implications of this process. Health resources have ultimately to be administered into the body to acquire meaning.

My next set of questions focus on a group of individuals and families in the central neighborhood of *Būlāq* on the eastern bank of the Nile. This is a five-hundred-year-old neighborhood well attached to the contemporary history of the whole city. Various aspects of this location and the reasons for choosing it are explained in the chapter on family life. *Būlāq* is a good place for my research because it is close to central Cairo, provided with multiple health resources, and has a socioeconomically diverse population. Further, it is a typical space where the family continues to play major roles.

I explore how different therapies are *experienced* within particular social relations. I choose to focus on the family because it is one of, if not the most significant social institution in the life of all persons of Cairo. The aim is to examine not only the meaning of health of the body but the *well-being* of the subjects involved. To use Lock's and Nguyen's terminology, I closely look at the "local biologies"; how the body is lived and experienced within its physical, social, moral, and political milieus. This is further illustrated by a cultural artifact called *'iḍḍaghṭ*, which is used by individuals from across the entire social scale to convey not mere physical pains but complex ones *felt* as related to moral, economic, and political conditions and circumstances that indirectly impinge on people's general sense of well-being. In Cairo that sense is deeply moral and political. I would argue that feeling well in Cairo is a traditional right that people would seek despite the evident material constraints. But these constraints have been excessively multiplied within the contemporary life conditions. The hallmark of life in Cairo in the mid-1990s when I did my research is a complex sense of distress and unhappiness summoning a whole range of disvalued emotions and feelings expressed by one single term called *'izza'al*. In brief, I would say during my research people of Cairo bitterly felt that the city was somehow "pressing them too hard."

My argument is that *'iḍḍaghṭ* proved to be expressive of an entirely non-medical but moral condition. It has been reworked as a means for social critique of the entire sociopolitical system that shaped and was shaping the individual subjectivities. I discuss the concept of the *subject* in terms of a local concept called *al-nafs* which may generally be translated to what Lock

(1987) calls "mindful body." *Al-nafs* is a Quranic term that points to a complex physic–psycho–socio–moral capacity rooted in the local tradition and responsible for mediating between individuals, their social surroundings, and the entire universe in this world and the life after. I ask the question, what are that roles played by this classical surviving notion in the present globalized, marketized, deeply divided, or even fragmented social life? The issue of transplanting body parts fits perfectly to pursue this question. In particular, I seek to identify the main authoritative institutions involved in constituting the discourse on the body in terms of *al-nafs*. I ask, who are the agents responsible for authoring the discourse on the body, are they in agreement? Are their ideas debated? What are the moral and political underpinnings of these debates? How would they look when placed in midst of those operating in everyday life and relating to my respondents?

This study is based on field research in Būlāq for two years (1995–1997). I was privileged to live in this great city, meet and visit families, build friendships, engage in public conversations, and follow public debates on various issues circulated by the national press, different television stations, the cinema, and others. My systematic ethnographic observations are mainly from *Būlāq*, which I initially approached from one of its most popular spaces: its cafés. With their chairs and tables placed inside as well as outside on the sidewalk they present an open invitation for walking and talking to visitors. They are operated by one or two men who serve *shīsha*, the water pipe for smoking sweetened tobacco, in addition to a whole variety of drinks including tea, coffee, and herb drinks such as fenugreek (*ḥilba*), hibiscus (*karkadaih*), anise (*yānsūn*), and mint (*na'nāᶜ*). All cafés are open for no less than twelve hours a day for men to relax, chat with friends, or play cards or dice. In much the same way as an English pub, the café is a meeting point to meet with friends for various purposes, including keeping up with the various affairs of the neighborhood, looking for new jobs, watching football matches on TV, and so forth. I used to be a smoker and admirer of the Egyptian *shīsha* and I participated in these activities before I talked to some men about their various private and public concerns. The beverages served are simultaneously used for various medicinal purposes and thus were useful for me to initiate casual chats with the men who were ready to explain what they knew about these traditional remedies.

Another aspect of space which had long fascinated me and which I always thought of as potentially very relevant to medical anthropological research in Egypt is the *mūlid* (pl. *mawālid*). This is a long-lived tradition of commemorating past Muslim mystic (*sūfi*) saints (*awliya*, sing. *wali*). The biggest *mūlid* in *Būlāq* is that of *al-Tarīqa al-Shāthiliyya* (the path of al-Shāthiliyya, named after the *tarīqa* leader *al-Sheikh al-Shāthili*).[2] Every year thousands of people from different parts of the country join the people of *Būlāq* to celebrate this occasion. They all use a large tent set up on the street next to the tomb of *al-Sheikh Salāmah*, the latest successor of *al-Sheikh al-Shāthili*. The tent hosts the main ritual of the *mūlid* called *zikr* (remembrance of God, the Prophet and the Sheikh), a collective chant and dance for men and women who stand separately in different sections of the tent.

Incidental events ignited my interest in engaging the life of people in Cairo. The first one included Sultan whom I met in a *mūlid*. Sultan was not religious, which is not uncommon among the *mūlid* goers. He was there for fun. I was there for personal interest, curiosity, and fun too. Sultan is from *Būlāq,* which is a major neighborhood of Cairo described in chapter 2. Most of my ethnographic fieldwork occurred in this neighborhood. Sultan introduced me to his family who then generously accepted that I visit them frequently. They introduced me to their family friends who lived in the area and well beyond. My research started and continued to follow a snowball methodology.

This method proved to be the best to learn about local lives with the least amount of control possible. I learned to further learn about their health and life experiences. Sultan was jobless at the time but he normally worked as a waiter on boat-restaurants docked by the Nile bank. Collecting health experiences from Sultan's family was crucial to learn key terms, concepts, feelings, and ways to maintain not necessarily health alone but the general sense of wellness in Cairo. Generally, this family generally belongs to lower income groups. All the adults of the family routinely complain of various kinds of pain resulting from problems characterizing their lives. The ways they utilize the available heath care resources however reveal a great repertoire of knowledge about various kinds of herb-based therapies and meditations to cure anxiety. These were managed at home and often under the supervision of women. They wouldn't be viewed as strictly medical. They are routinely practiced during prayers, food, and drinks. One needs to mention something that hurts for others to start providing advice and help in no time. This family belongs to the largest economic class in Egypt. Life within this class is generally characterized by great sense of empathy and mutual support. Illness and pain are very special cases where these feelings occur in spontaneous manners.

Away from the house the family would trust modern biomedical therapies the most. Their first choice is to see specialized physicians operating privately. But these are not always trusted due to current developments that lead to the marketization of the health care system. The general sense in Cairo is that medical care has become a business sought mainly for profit. Many people have health insurance from the government but none of them would trust the governmental services because they use dated and cheaply maintained equipment that are run by poorly paid personnel who also may also be underqualified. In all cases, most of the persons included in my research would not be satisfied with using physical therapies alone. Their major concern is with life as a whole. What is generally known as spiritual or belief-based therapies from supplication, to visiting healers, are done routinely in the times of illness and in daily life.

Generally, people in Cairo very highly regard peace, relaxation, and tranquility as preconditions for good health. The expression of being in "*kuwayyis*" is one of many that express this value and desire. Naglaa' was one of the women I met because she visited a hospital I was using to conduct interviews on *'iḍḍaghṭ*. She suffered from various pains and aches that took her to several physicians and healers. But she could not believe any of the diagnoses offered including *'iḍḍaghṭ*, irregular heartbeat, weak blood, malnutrition, among others. She would assert that none of these is true and "even if they were so, I would recover very quickly if I manage to have a sense of peace in my home among my husband and many children." I view aspect of health care as a *trope* (Good, M., Hyde, Pinto, and B. Good 2008: 3) connecting issues of wellness, illness, and death to the conditions and issues characterizing the community surrounding the subjects and society at large.

Throughout my stay in Cairo I met with many doctors, nurses, and officials working in hospitals, private clinics, pharmacies, herb shops, and dispensaries sponsored by local mosques in *Būlāq* and other parts of the city. Initially, I visited these facilities with people from the families I got to know in *Būlāq*. In these visits, some of the health practitioners were unwilling to give detailed information about their practices or about the work of their organizations. The ones who are working for clinics sponsored by mosques and Islamic organizations are involved in opposition politics and thus were especially discreet. They have to censor the information they release to outsiders fearing that they are somehow connected to the government. Others who are working for the governmental health facilities are keen to present somewhat of an "official" version of their practice. In addition, many doctors were keen to present their views in highly standardized medical terms. Whether that is for professional reasons or because they wanted to avoid the social or political aspects of health care, the result was the same: little informality and limited opportunity to know their views about their daily lives and work conditions.

I was led to learn most of my knowledge about the informal dimensions of life after I accidently met Magdy who is a physician and social activist. I first met Magdy when he was giving a public talk to students on the significance of traditional healing as essential components of the contemporary health care scenery of Cairo. In the subsequent days Magdy introduced me to major hospitals and practitioners and assisted my interviewing patients in various medical facilities. He did that for no return because we became friends. During those visits Magdy described much of his views that confirm the above thoughts. He was trained as a physician in Cairo University. Shortly after his graduation he witnessed how dysfunctional the health system was not because of the lack of expertise or equipment. The main problem was that the entire system was inherently focused on the physical aspects of wellness: "It did not pay attention to issues of poverty, social justice, equality, urban organization, education, and many other aspects" that for Magdy are essential elements to have a sense of well-being. Shortly after leaving his job as a physician Magdy joined several nongovernmental organizations before he turns to journalism. It was Magdy who led me to pay further attention to ways larger issues of political economy indirectly were experienced and felt by individuals and families.

SOCIETY IN HEALTH AND ILLNESS

Meanings of health and life are manufactured in spaces much wider than those represented by single therapies devised for particular complaints. They are shaped by discourses of power produced by centralized institutions. As such, they can be viewed as indices for studying the workings of the apparatuses responsible for running the existing relations of power. From among these I am particularly concerned with the family, the clinic, the law, religion, and, most significantly, the state. My argument is that all these are constituted by the country's long-standing traditions where health is embedded in matrix including meanings of optimism, integrity, harmony, and justice, next of course to physical fitness.

Central to this study is the distinction between health and medicine. I view the former as referring to *optimum states* characterizing life as a whole. It is dependent on the availability of favorable physical, social, *and* moral conditions. Implied by the term "optimum" is the idea that health is a measure of a socially acceptable *balance* between various conditions of life. Thus, health status is an index measuring the goodness of life. Most relevant to this study is the idea that health status implies both a human right and a social obligation. This is a rather moral aspect of health central to the Arabic term *Ṣiḥḥah*, which describes health together with a set of other meanings concerned with being right, correct, coherent, and, most significantly, *just* or *fair*. Medicine is a different thing. It refers primarily to the practical means to treat particular physical and mental conditions. Most significant, it is a resource. The knowledge it employs is practical but value-laden. Issues of justice, ethical integrity, and aesthetics are constantly used in evaluating the results of medical care. I am concerned with this complex knowledge as an integrated whole that includes no separation between the body and mind, the real and unreal, the individual and social, the objective and subjective, the visible and invisible. This knowledge is ultimately represented by the subjects involved. This perspective is long established in social studies of health care (see Young 1982, Csordas 1993, and Lock and Farquhar 2007) and based on compelling ethnographic studies and even recent concepts such as "local biology" and "postcoloniality."

LOCAL BIOLOGIES, SUBJECTIVITY IN A POSTCOLONIAL CONTEXT

In this section I describe concepts central to description and analysis of my study. First I discuss the notion of "local biologies" that are shaped by both physical and subjective factors and mechanisms. They constitute unique living physical forms or "experienced bodies" so to speak. In this context the notion of the subject and subjectivity play major roles. In the present world society these exist and are shaped within postcolonial sociopolitical milieus very relevant to Egypt in the past and present. My study focuses on one traditional notion called *al-nafs* which I view as the cultural space for shaping local subjectivities. Each part of my study is an illustration of various aspects of this complex notion of *al-nafs*. In brief, this is a relational concept that could be understood as a "local biology," a space for shaping subjectivity illustrating the postcolonial condition experienced differentially across the whole society.

Local biology is a concept developed by Lock and Nguyen (2010) to challenge the assumed universality of the human body underlying biomedicine. It refers to patterned variations in subjective bodily experiences ensuing from mutually shaping physical, cultural, and psychological factors specific to particular historical environments. Local biologies are reproduced through material and cultural mechanisms distinctive to specific historical milieus. Lock and Nguyen discuss four themes to illustrate this notion: menopause, *Kuru* (a mysterious epidemic among the Fore of New Guinea), the relationship between racism and low birth weights, and the theories for explaining HIV. The four cases illustrate how biological differentiation is intricately associated with particular sociocultural and psychological dynamics.

The case of menopause explains the significance of local biology and its relevance to my study. The authors use this condition to show that differences in individual bodily experiences at the end of menstruation "must be understood as local entanglements among historical and cultural activities, technoscientific interventions, and the biology of individual aging" (Lock and Nguyen 2010: 83). In the case of Europe, the United States, and Australia the dominant "local biology" has been one of a disease-like condition; the concept of menopause was fused with the end of menstrual cycling. It was then enmeshed with medical and pharmaceutical interests to manage and supply it with curative drugs that may limit its symptoms (*ibid*: 85).

Then authors oppose the claim that menopause was a result of longer life expectancy due to improved health conditions. They offer a more sophisticated explanation based on comparative studies between the United States, Canada, and Japan. They note that Japan has had a category (*Kônenki*) that is partly similar to those predating menopause in English. But the meanings of the terms concerned are not identical. Further, the Japanese language does not offer term's that *uniquely* describe hot flashes. The terms available are translations of foreign ones. As such, women's experiences in Japan were only occasionally similar to those of North America. The best way to describe them therefore is to use terms offered by the local biology resulting from measurable physiological changes mediated by subjective experiences as well as the reporting of symptoms whose biological pathways may sometimes be poorly understood. In the words of Lock and Nguyen "local biologies are artifacts—snapshots frozen in time of ceaseless biosocial differentiation" (90). Here we are speaking about a "real" phenomenon taking place to every woman. The issue though is the diverse way such phenomena are produced, construed, and circulated by and among various actors occupying different social roles. More significant, is the way these phenomena are known and intervened in.

Local biologies are reproduced by *mechanisms* evident in specific situations occurring within social and political arrangements. In the case of menopause, mechanisms include physiological processes running within Japanese environments with distinctive diets, and subjectively experienced rules, values, norms as well sense of aesthetics and well-being. Mechanisms then are physical processes embedded within ethnic–environmental variables contributing to the production of health and sickness-engendering agents. These mechanisms may not be singular or composed of unitary operations or agents. Several mechanisms may coexist and not be always in agreement as in the case of *Kuru* or HIV. Several theories have been offered to explain the last two epidemics. Each theory was entangled with sets of social, cultural and professional interest and paradigms. The resulting mechanisms were trans-local and even global.

The term *subject* is used as verb in descriptions of situations, conditions, or events marked with some sense of passivity to presumably external forces. In addition, it is used to distinguish between "subjects of an authoritarian regime on the one hand and consenting or self-legislating citizens" on the other. Subjectivity too contrasts with objectivity or socially compromised approaches to common facts constructed as exterior to individual experiences (Rorty 2007: 35). Subjective feelings and positions do not always exist in peace with those regarded objectives. The latter are viewed as neutral because they have been agreed upon by a majority of voices. Cultural ethnographers have been among one of the most sensitive social scientists toward subjective views of the communities they studied. Among those there are researchers who insist on representing local communities in local terms. They would keep their intervention to the least amount possible.

An example about Egypt is Watson's ethnography *Women in the City of the Dead* (1992) that includes stories told by women in the first person. But that is the only ethnography about Egypt concerned with this kind of anthropology. Moreover, other examples of subjectivity studies have hardly been concerned with the issue of local biologies discussed above. Currently however there is an agenda to focus on subjectivity justified by methodological and epistemic reasons. It is also motivated by moral and ethical sensibilities and guided by practical purposes. From a purely practical vantage point, personal ideas and feeling as well as dietary habits and rules ultimately contribute to shaping the material reality as discussed above. Second, curative and healing activities that address pain and suffering often require active participation of the patients in the therapeutic process. "Some medical ethicists argue that an 'I–Thou' dialogic sensibility that responds to the voice of the subject evokes a constructive partnership in healing: it elicits attentiveness, engagement, and sensitivity from medical practitioners and active cooperation by patients" (Rorty 2007: 47). The general historic survey that Rorty provides for the notion of the subject confirms that all the major Christian and philosophic traditions are now represented in anthropological writings. Those include the power of the confessional expression developed by Augustine, the authenticity of the unmediated experience of pain and suffering Ignatius, the Cartesian epistemic privilege of the introspective reflection of the self, the origins of the fictional idea of the self described by Hume, the egalitarian direction of the rights of individual autonomy by Rousseau, and the dialogical "we" of self-positing "I" philosophized by Sartre and Fichte (Rorty 2007: 48). One major theme that has returned to anthropological discourse is that of the repressed subject. I think much of the current subjectivities should be understood within local, regional, and globalized relations of power and hegemony responsible for shaping conditions of life in postcolonial societies like Egypt.

In order to appreciate cultural artifacts like local biologies we should pay attention to the elements and mechanisms employed in the constitution of the *subject* and the various forms that subjection takes in diverse milieus. Furthermore, we need to examine how lives of individuals, families, and communities are affected by large-scale political and economic forces associated with the building of national economy within the context of globalization for example. These effects should be narrated in local cultural terms including in particular those concerned with the subject and subjectivity. In my research this concept is called *al-nafs* and I will discuss it after the following brief note.

How does subjectivity look in context of postcoloniality? First the term *culture* itself is problematized especially when used to describe disordered experience investigated by social scientists. These researchers are brought into conversation with those studying political subjectivity and postcolonial theorizing. Further, detailed ethnographic studies are inserted within larger literary and theoretical studies that are often regarded as unrelated to everyday experience (Good et al. 2008). In other words, the notion of the postcolonial benefits the study of subjectivity because it helps articulate it in terms circulated within larger fields of power that ultimately impinge on the lives of the studied communities although they may not be readily discernible in their everyday circumstances. Most interesting is that the notion of the postcolonial helps bring the psychological into the political and vice versa. Colonial and postcolonial relations of power in this context consist in a *trope* construed in literary rather than purely scientific terms. The postcolonial is presented as a "specter often present but in only ghostly forms in current anthropological writings on subjectivity" (Good et al. 2008: 5).

The postcolonial perspective points to an era that profoundly influenced the contemporary society of Egypt. It helps focus on the way institutions have been modeled after their European counterparts and continued to operate, interact, and develop within a hierarchy that placed them in the most powerful positions vis-à-vis the continuing traditional institutions. An order was created to define what was rational and what was not, what was systematic and what was chaotic, what was to be included and what was to be excluded. That order was not brought in by European hands alone. Egyptian significant thinkers, reformers, and practitioners have participated too (Mitchell 1991). It is necessary to stress that that order was not substantially altered upon the erection of the nation-state that has supposedly driven the colonial forces off the country's borders. In place was already set an array of institutional structures along with a sense of order deciding on the basic principles of almost all fields of life. Of course that order included a discourse responsible for pathologizing and exclusionary. But these tasks were of course carried out in terms adapted to local tradition including of course those of Islam and Arabic.

Similarly, my position is that human biology is inevitably a social and material artifact. The various ways it is perceived, felt, understood, represented, and intervened provide an avenue and index for social life. Our physical sense of well-being and feelings are ultimately inseparable from the technologies employed to describing, modifying, or representing it. My present study tackles various conditions of the human body as artifacts lived by the subjects involved; "life" which ultimately is the equivalent to the term "local biology" suggested by Lock and Nguyen. In local terms life is referred to by the term *al-nafs*. My argument is that communities of my study have local biologies resulting from the physical conditions as subjectively experienced within of respective local social-cultural environments. The health practices described are reproduced through mechanisms composed of the material and physiological processes articulated in terms of and in reference to ideas and feelings distinguishing local subjectivities.

AL-NAFS: THE CULTURAL SPACE FOR SUBJECTIVITY

In this vein comes the local distinction between the soul (*al-nafs*, pl. *nufūs*) and the body (*al-jism*). These two categories do not form a dichotomy either. *Al-nafs* is a multifaceted term used to denote a great variety of spiritual and physical states of life. In standard Arabic it means the person. In the Egyptian dialect it simultaneously connotes meanings of the mind, emotional pain, the appetite, giving birth, envy, desire, price, and many others. It is an ancient term that survived in Islamic tradition as a relational *(mushtarak)* concept referring to *al-'insān* (human) who is neither a body (*badan*) nor a spirit or mind *(jinn or rūh)* but a person or soul. According to a very influential twelfth-century scholar, al-Ghazali, *al-nafs* is the core within which different interdependent aspects of what we know as human are constituted (al-Ghazali 2008). This same notion of human has been carried over by contemporary scholars. Most notable is Mohammed Qutb who is one of the most influential authors on the subject. A careful examination of one major book by Qutb reveals that *al-nafs* is conceptualized in ways guided by Islamic traditions but very aware of the modern science of psychology.[3]

In the last hundred years or so *al-nafs* has also been used by modern psychologists to mean the psyche. Psychology in Arabic is called *'ilm al-nafs* (the science of the soul). This concept has adapted to carry multiple meanings deriving from contemporaneous traditions responsible for constructions of life and death. It is reproduced as an amalgam in diverse contexts. The relevance of this concept to my study will be clear in the subsequent chapters when its roles in describing life, health, and illness are discussed in contexts of the living culture and issues of social relations of power in the contemporary society of Egypt. It will be clear that *al-nafs* is host to emotions, beliefs, ideas, and dispositions that contribute to shaping the physical and mental characteristics of individuals and groups. Most crucial to my study is the observation that *al-nafs* is a *precondition* to the existence of the body and the person in life and death. Therefore, it is not possible to access the body, either conceptually or practically, apart from various aspects of *al-nafs*.

Modern social science based on the Cartesian split between the body and mind falls short of coping with these multiple meanings. Much still has to be done to develop theoretical approaches for appreciating human life as an integrated unity including society. In the existing literature, *al-nafs* is very close to Lock and Scheper-Hughes's mindful body but closer to MacIntyre's notion of a unified virtuous subject (1987: 206). It can also be approximated to important aspects of the notion of habitus developed first by Mauss (1970 [1935]) and adopted later by Bourdieu (1998). What matters here is to emphasize that we are before a unique traditional concept developed into a new form in response to changing conditions of social life. The best way to explore it is to describe how it is variously experienced in everyday life characterized by plurality and change, which is discussed at several points in this book and mainly in chapter 1. In the context of *al-nafs*, individuals are represented not as skin-bound bodies possessing an autonomous and active agency. They are *nāss* (humans), *persons* who possess rights and fulfill duties and perform roles attached to a sense of identity, aesthetics, and virtues.

In practice, what matters are the complex subjective experiences. Life occurs in diverse social contexts that contribute to the formation of what Lock and Farquhar (2007) call the *lived body*.[4] The latter includes forms of the "body proper" adapted to a variety of practical contexts. The lived body therefore points to open-ended, dynamic, and plural human experiences of carnality that are historically contingent, shaped and inspired by culture, and diversely regulated by social relations of power. The lived body also includes the mind and is not one of its contrastive categories. It is historically variable and dependent on long-standing traditions and local biologies.

Various meanings of *al-nafs* are explored and discussed in the course of this study by viewing individual respondents as persons or rather subjects as explained above. Their consciousness however is mediated through experienced embodiment, which is inherently social. This is why the individuals included in my study are situated within the relations most significant to them, their families, and society at large. Their experiences, however, are simultaneously political, subjective, objective, discursive, narrative, and physical. All these aspects are culturally and historically specific. They are adaptable and thus ought to be examined using the local mutable terms offered by local discourses. This is the reason I examine health-related practices in texts, conversations, films, and other media. Human experience is multifaceted and necessitates opening a domain of experience that is "subjective and objective, carnal and conscious, observable and legible" (*ibid*: 10).

Chapter 4 is included in this book because it presents different ways of imagining the body in unique, recently emerging states of being including brain death and life after death. Second, this book is ultimately about life and politics on life represented by the notion of the subject in the context of *al-nafs*. Organ donation is a process of transferring forms of life in the form of vital organs. The transference is essentially a process of exchange that reveals meanings central to the local ethical issues. Third, this chapter brings society into the body and the body into society including of course the kinds of subjectivities at work. Fourth, the range of ideas, opinions, and feelings expressed on the debate on organ donation illustrates that the notion of culture is not a given but a question; the fact that all aspects of donation are debated illustrates this fact very well. Fifth, there is a very interesting link between ethics and subjectivity in Islamic communities (Moosa 2005). This link is essential for practices to be socially meaningful in Muslim communities. The relevance of this issue will be evident when I discuss the book as a whole in chapter 5. Finally, the debates take place in a society that has been colonized and then ruled by nation-state run by local elites. It has been excessively globalized and subjected to an encroaching market that contributed to the commodification of social life. The debates in this context provide an index reflecting the range of attitudes, positions, and subjective views and the way they are debated and changed.

The materials upon which this chapter is based are almost totally from the press. During the process of collecting them I was living in Cairo. I engaged in discussions on the theme with several officials including most significantly the head of the doctors' syndicate and administrators of governmental hospitals, and political activists concerned with the ethical and moral aspects of these controversial questions. I also met with people who received organs. These data certainly helped me interpret data from the press.

The above discussion on subjectivity throws a sense of dissatisfaction about the capacity of the notion of culture to describe the complex human condition in the present society. As a means of provocation it suggests to use the "postcolonial" instead of culture. It brings together specific issues critical to contemporary society not included in the too general concept of culture. Issues of violence represented by theft of human organs and aggravated by class divisions protected by a postcolonial corrupt state nourishing an economic system resting on crony capitalism that privileges a few while impoverishing the majority of the population under the auspices of complacent if not colluding legal system is best represented by the term *postcolonial*. These are the conditions under which the subjects of my study live and have to struggle in explicit and implicit ways. The theme of organ transplantation illustrates these conditions perfectly because it shows how they operate on the most intimate aspect of the people's lives—their bodies and their lives as well as those of their beloved. The questions I discuss in chapter 4 and this whole book in general are not about medicine and health, although these are my main empirical fields. My inquiry is about the politico-ethical aspects of living within the increasingly aggressive environment of Cairo dominated by a free market and corrupt state apparatus.

MEDICAL PLURALITY FROM COMPARATIVE PERSPECTIVES

Health care has long been viewed as a social and cultural practice. The assumption is that the practices labeled as "medical" operate and are operated upon within the general field of subjectivity. My research confirms the idea of "local biology" discussed in this book. An endlessly recurrent observation throughout my research would occur in so many vignettes. These would include men and women who would speak about their pains by referring to their concerns about their children, or the polluted air in the city, or the increasingly demoralized society due to increased pressures and inability to cope with these. These complex narratives would turn the theme of health and wellness into a trope summarizing all complex efforts to accommodate all the surrounding conditions. The metaphors and stories narrated cannot be accounted for by one single component of the health care system in Cairo. Medical pluralism therefore proves to be relevant and enjoying a great explanatory capacity in this context (cf. Greenwood et al. 1988 and Mullings 1986).

The concept of medical pluralism provided a tool for earlier research on the social aspects of health care practices. It refers to contexts characterized by the availability of several kinds of medical traditions. In countries like the United States where the medical system has long been seen as entirely based on therapies collectively called biomedicine, the use of these therapies occurs in a "a pluralistic network of different kinds of physicians, dentists, clinical psychologists, chiropractors, health food experts, yoga teachers, spirit curers, druggists, Chinese herbalists, and so on" (Leslie 1976: 357). China also presents a more diverse and complex case. There, biomedicine has always had to coexist with the country's long-standing therapeutic traditions that correspond to the nation's social structures. As these traditions were institutionalized and reorganized throughout the last century they were reorganized into a system of therapy to interact and change with incoming biomedicine

(Leslie 1980: 191). Although influential in distinctive ways, the two traditions keep a relative degree of interdependence. In India, medicines rooted in the Ayurvedic and the Islamic-Yunani (Greek) traditions existed side by side and developed their own institutionalized structures next to the biomedical ones (Zimmerman 1978; Banerji 1985, 1981). The coexistence implies processes of interaction and change (Foster 1984).

Social scientists' use of the concept of medical pluralism was predominantly aimed at describing "health seeking behaviors" (Foster 1987), which sometimes involved *choosing* between different therapies (Davis 1988) or healers (Amarasingham, 1980; Heggenhougen 1980) in order to maximize the therapeutic benefits from the resources available. Some used the concept of "hierarchy of resort" (Lane and Millar 1987; Ramanocci-Ross 1969) to emphasize that different resources are unequally ranked in terms of the social values ascribed to them. These and other studies aim at improving the utilization of health resources (see, for example, Nichter 1980). Some suggested that this improvement could be achieved if traditional healers are included in the biomedical establishment. This was an attempt to overcome health dilemmas in the developing world.[5]

Despite the large number of these studies, little attempt has been made to study the sociopolitical implications of the *composite forms* of therapy, which result from combining elements belonging to different traditions. For example, the relationship between the healing experiences that take place in the context of this area of interactivity overlap on one hand, and the cultural order on the other, has not been sufficiently developed as an independent field for investigation (cf. Comaroff 1980). In this vein, early anthropological accounts presented aspects of interaction between different medical resources. In his widely cited study, "The Quest for Therapy: Medical Pluralism in Lower Zaire," Janzen (1978) demonstrates that people merge biomedical therapies and their traditional and religious or spiritual therapeutic practices. The implication of this process is that medical systems are articulated methods of explanation and treatment. This articulation is not embodied in the conceptual frameworks of the medical systems, but rather in the *practice* of these cultural constructs. The following quote from Janzen illustrates this idea.

> Most therapy managing groups were desirous of continuing specific physical treatment, preferably in a Western medical institution, until the patient had recovered. But their conviction that less tangible social and mystical causes had intervened obliged them to intersperse visits to dispensary or hospital with visits to banganga, who could deal with anger, to convene kinship councils to settle conflicts, or to see prophets for council in life crisis decisions (Janzen 1978: 226).[6]

Another, early attempt to examine this relationship is Leslie (1976) who presents the contemporary health practices of India under several forms that originated in the Ayurvedic medicine rooted in the Sanskrit classic texts, and the Yunani medicine rooted in the classic Arabic texts. He notes that throughout the centuries the interaction between different healers had produced a syncretic medicine of traditional culture, which evolved among learned practitioners from the thirteenth to the nineteenth centuries. In addition, these traditions have been professionalized. They subsequently assimilated many elements from cosmopolitan medical knowledge and institutions, which had been implanted and supported by the colonial state and subsequently continued by the postcolonial one. In addition, India contains a great variety of "homeopathic medical practices, learned magico-religious curing and folk medical practices" (*ibid*: 359). Within such complex structure of medical care Leslie writes that a diverse popular culture of healing emerged as the institutions of mass society grew along with the "industrial production of medicine, advertising and the school system" (*ibid*). Syncretism continued, and composite forms of therapy proliferated and combined humoral concepts with germ theory, and the vitamins with hot and cold foods. This practice

> combines the humoral concepts of hot and cold foods with concepts of vitamins; traditional physiological concepts with the germ theory of disease; popular astrology and religion with faith in modern science and technology. It utilizes patent medicines and drugs from modern chemotherapy, along with industrially prepared Ayurvedic, Yunani and homeopathic medications (*ibid*).[7]

The continued coexistence of medical practices based on disparate social, religious, and ontological assumptions subsequently led anthropologists to conclude that medical pluralism may be linked to "multiplicity of competing interests or power groups" (Lewis and Frankel 1989: 30), or to the "replication of similar and competing organizations in the same institutional sphere" (*ibid*). Pluralism as "opposed to monism" thus "rejects the world as unity" (*ibid*: 3). This formulation is directly related to my study. I view healing as a social and political process based on religious, legal, and moral ideas as well as purely medical ones. I will return to this idea in the section on methods.

For now I use the notion of *medical pluralism* because it helps to examine interactions between different therapeutic traditions. I would like to draw attention to the fact that in the present world of juxtaposed cultures new forms of therapy associated with novel awareness of the body emerge due to simultaneous use of different elements rooted in diverse methods and life philosophies. I suggest analyzing these as "composite form"—amalgams of different elements meant to treat particular ailments. These forms are produced because of pure practical needs. However, these are defined as objects and subjects based on philosophical and ideological positions. The latter are hardly, if ever, uniform or homogeneous. The interaction between them often results in discourses animated by conflicting material interests. All this occurs within institutional structures in search of appropriate and effective actions. Such choices imply taking a position over debated concepts and values. They also imply taking positions over debated interventions. Different ideological positions possess disparate amounts of power, whether material or otherwise.

However, these positions sound abstract. How can they be observed? The concept of *therapeutic process* refers to all actions and processes intended to preserve the health of the individual and the integrity of the social group is useful in this regards. I hold that different ideological positions illustrate the continuing functions of medicine as both a means for social control and resistance, which can be observed in the ways diseases are constructed and represented by people's narratives. Taking pluralism into consideration it is possible to compare the way different concepts operate in different situations rather than grand structures with little relevance to particular individual events or illness episodes. It also enables us to study how conceptual distinctions are themselves subject to critique from those involved in therapeutic and other practices.

But what does happen to "local biologies" or *al-nafs* in contexts of medical pluralism? The latter concept has long been invested in the material notion of life and thus occupied the center of the originally western biomedical paradigm. Simultaneously, it has played key roles in comparative studies of health care systems supposedly based on cultural relativism that aimed at developing general theories. I suspect such reliance has caused these studies to be in the service of systems focused on the body as the main object of health care. They may have hindered the development of a general theory for the comparative study of health care systems by tacitly privileging particular assumptions of single systems (cf. Scheper-Hughes and Lock 1987, Lock 1993, Farquhar and Lock 2007). I think using the concept of *al-nafs* provides a holistic view basic to the entire anthropological discourse. This notion is directly related to the notion of the *soul*, which is the closest term to translate the cultural notion of the person that plays a major role in explaining not merely the occurrence of illness but the realization of health and well-being.

The notion of *al-nafs* also provides grounds to understand *nafsanah* that means to desire to possess material and immaterial assets. Second, many of the complaints uttered by the subjects included in this study are explained by the term *hāla nafsiyaa,* which means that the cause of pain is an uncomfortable state of the soul. *Al-nafs* therefore offers a terrain in which we can speak about the body in moral terms that address major problems afflicting not merely discrete individual bodies but rather the entire fabric of the social body as a whole or the very logic upon which it is based as subjectively experienced. Examples illustrating this idea will be discussed in the chapter concerned with family life, chapter 2, and *'iḍḍaghṭ*, chapter 3. Third, and most significantly, this notion includes the physical body and offers a completely different ground to speak of a spectrum of nuanced feelings and senses of the world than offered by the term *embodiment*. This spectrum provides a terrain to speak about life in relational and holistic ambitions; it enables speakers to include the physical, psychological, social, and politico-moral aspects of life all at once. Finally, and given that the researcher is also *ensouled*, it offers an opportunity for intersubjective interpretations of the observed practices.

Life and well-being and health and happiness are socioeconomic resources. In stratified societies they, like the therapies used to maintain and promote them, are unequally appropriated. They are organized to serve society's different relations of power. Health in the holistic sense of the term means life, which is all that is implied by the notion of *al-nafs*—a unit resulting from the combination of body and mind. This morality-focused notion is tied to the world in which it lives in multiple ways. It has the potential to mirror and accommodate the existence of the universe in its entirety. The constructions of the *sūfis* are only extreme examples. In Islam all humans have this capacity. The difference between different persons is only in degree.

Al-nafs can subject the social world as well as the individual it represents to continuous moral evaluations. Curiously, it is also believed to be entirely shapeable by society; humans are born completely blank and their souls are given content by their social milieu. I argue that *al-nafs* is a core component of a moral discourse invested in shaping subjectivity concerned with the production of social rights and desire.

Al-nafs in Islamic tradition primarily performs three main functions. It leads persons to commit sins (*al-nafs al-ammarah bissou'*). Second, it prohibits them from doing so because it sustains a sense of blame for wrongdoings (*al-nafs al-lawwamah*). The result is a precarious sense of balance between the sinful *nafs* and the blaming *nafs* that may result in another sense of content characterized by tranquility and peace. The result is conditioned by fulfilling moral requirements of being fair and just. These three functions mean that *al-nafs* is a state of being dependent on moral performance shared and thus subject for social evaluation.

POLITICAL ECONOMY AND HEALTH CARE

The present society is market-based. Consumer culture operates to sustain desires and generate new ones. Simultaneously, the fulfillment of these is constructed as a basic human right. Therefore *al-nafs* is perceived as a host of rightfully deserved needs and desires; it plays a major role in evaluating the health status and judging the adequacy of relevant social services. The latter are not merely medicinal: more profoundly, they include all practices aiming to sustain and improve living conditions. In this sense *al-nafs* is simultaneously a means to *feel* and represent living conditions, a moral measure to evaluate the conditions in the light of the health status achieved, and, most significantly, an agent to demand fulfilling whatever is needed and desired for a good living. In this endeavor *al-nafs* relies upon ideas, emotions, and feelings conceived in a relational manner.

A good ethnographic example to illustrate this point is Paul Farmer's (1988) article on the syndrome of *move san/lèt gate* among women in rural Haiti. Farmer's general interest is in interpreting corporeal complaints in relation to nonbodily experiences. He rests his analysis on theoretical formulations that connect the physical, social, and political body through the study of emotions. Such a formulation transcends the classic and long criticized division between the mind and the body. The article is focused on one folk sickness called *move san* (bad blood) common among women in rural Haiti. This syndrome supposedly starts in the blood and later manifests itself in other parts of the body including the head, limbs, skin, and uterus. Most serious among the consequences of the syndrome is called *lèt gate*, which refers to the corruption of the milk of lactating mothers. *Move san* is thus frequently cited as a motive for early weaning that leads to damaging effects on the infants' health. The syndrome is explained in emotional terms, which fit the kind of complex and intimate relations and feelings it involves. Farmer writes, "the significance of the syndrome lies in the fact that social problems and their psychological sequelae usually are designated as the causes of the somatically experienced disorder" (Farmer 1988: 63). By examining the ways the syndrome is explained by the afflicted women, the healers, he concludes that this complex syndrome is caused by "malignant emotions—anger born of interpersonal strife, shock, grief, chronic worry, and other affects perceived as potentially harmful" (*ibid*). Most interesting in Farmer's study is that it illustrates that the different explanations belong to a field entirely different from the one presented to the modern village physician. The reason behind the clustering of the interpretations of the *move san* lies in the fact that

> *Move san/lèt gate* is a "public health problem" in an unaccustomed sense: an illness with a public meaning. When a whole village knows the participants and follows the course of treatment, a case of *move san/lèt gate* serves as a stage on which social and psychological problems (mistreatment of pregnant or lactating women, for example) *can be aired* (Farmer 1988: 74, emphasis added).

Then Farmer argues that "Body fluids like milk and blood are perceived as especially sensitive to 'malignant' emotions; disorders involving them can therefore be seen as '*barometers*' of disturbances in the social field" (Farmer 1988: 75, *emphasis added*).

Farmer's analysis is a good illustration of the issue of "somatization" I criticize above. He views *move san* as a complex phenomenon encompassing all the complex life aspects indicated by the patients, for example in the previous quotation. These aspects obviously call for a new conceptualization of human pain, different from that implied by the word "soma," which again sets the body apart from the mind. My idea is that there should be a new term that may involve the body, but also emphasizes the other aspects stressed by Farmer as a cornerstone in the patients' explanations of *move san*, namely, their emotions. Finally, however, Farmer argues that if meaning-centered interpretive approaches are to make sense, their results should be linked to the political economic structures within which they, and the narratives which form their basis, occur (Farmer 1988: 76).

In addition, I think the political economic perspective allows viewing the meanings involved as debatable rather than consensual. It views the therapeutic process as involving various ways of reasoning that may be in conflict. As we will see, more often than not, these ways are associated with social groups occupying different positions in the power structure of society. The adoption of this approach, however, should not necessarily lead to an authoritative position that claims the ability to distinguish particular knowledge as "true" in contrast to other knowledge that might be called "mystified" or simply false (cf. Young 1982). Such a position, I contend, would do no less than reproduce the classic rationalist positions that once viewed modern science as the only way that could produce "true" knowledge (cf. Good 1995: 56–62). In contrast, a far more productive way to examine medicine and medical care, I think, is to juxtapose different kinds of knowledge and explore the ways in which certain points of view become more powerful than others. This would require situating the different views within the power structure of society. It would also require us to take into account the fact that these views are operating and interacting within localized political economic structures encompassed by the capitalist world system.

This approach is more suitable for the study of contemporary medical practices in Egypt, which have long been described as being far from monolithic or uniform (see Morsy 1978, 1980; Inhorn 1996: 49–77).[8] Central to my study is the observation that medical practices frequently rely on multiple medical and nonmedical measures to realize physical and social healing. Even when single therapies are used, as happens sometimes in my study, the larger process of healing is embedded in a complex array of processes involving religious and moral concepts and ways of reasoning. These processes connect the remedies in question to the traditions and history of the people who use and maintain them. By their practice and use of them, the subjects involved embody their cultural memory. The meanings attached to the therapies can change as a result of the different, and at times conflicting, material interests and ideological orientations of various social groups. When viewed through the perspective of medical pluralism such a situation leads to a plethora of therapeutic forms based on constantly varying social, cultural, and psychological circumstances. To study this diversification we need to view medicine as reproduced along with and in other domains including, for example, religion, the law, and morality. These ideas have led my study to be "multi-sited" (Marcus and Fischer 1986).

The political economy approach adequately emphasizes the notion of inequity in health care, which is enforced by the dominant social relations. The proponents of this perspective include people working in different disciplines such as public health and sociology of health. For these, what matters most are the unequal statuses of different therapeutic systems (Elling 1981) and the hegemonic power of biomedicine (Myntti 1981).[9] Baer, Singer, and Johnson (1986) present a programmatic paper that illustrates that different medical systems are organized in a hierarchical manner. By hierarchy they mean that the therapies of these systems are unequal in status and perhaps efficacy. The authors explain the hierarchy in terms of "levels," perhaps to indicate the element of inequality between different "systems" of therapy. The top level in this hierarchy, according to the authors, is called the "macro-social level." It encompasses plural medical systems in which modern biomedicine "enjoys a dominant status over heterodox and ethnomedical practices" (*ibid*: 96, see also Singer 1990; Morsy 1990; McKinlay 1985: 1–9).[10] Next is what the authors call the "intermediate level," which includes modern biomedicine and its administrative apparatus. The micro level involves the healer and/or healer-patient interaction. It also includes the patients and their support networks.

This approach highlights aspects of social conflict and change that are observable in medical practice. Such processes have been analyzed across regional (Heggenhougen 2000: 1172), national, and international (Morsy 1993) levels.[11] Forces operating at these "levels," all the authors working in this tradition would agree, are jointly impinging on the lives in localized communities.

> While many still identify with, and live most of their lives within the confines of, small, local communities, these are no longer untouched wholes, or "untainted" villages. The overwhelming forces of globalization . . . and of what has long been recognized as "commerciogenic" pathologizing forces of capitalism

> out of control . . . are facts of life, not only in urban centers, but as insidious also in the local settings that anthropologists know so well (Heggenhougen 2000: 1172).

Within such globalized contexts, the continuation of varying different resources came to be ascribed to *acts of exclusion* implicit in the discourse of biomedicine (Heggenhougen 1987: 48–49, emphasis mine). In particular, within social systems where biomedicine enjoys a dominant role in shaping health perceptions, significant aspects of life have long been neglected. For example, facts such as those with which individuals live and the way they identify their problems in close reference to problems and prospects experienced with and by their families have been left out of the concern of the mainstream biomedical establishment (*ibid*).

These views are not without problems. First, much of what is written within this approach has been rather prescriptive and assertive but lacking in substantive examples (Comaroff 1980). It has been based on preconceived ideas about social change presumably conditioned or determined by material forces. This determinism, I would argue, and the way it is distinguished is an expression of the by-now-sufficiently criticized split between the mind and the body (see Scheper-Hughes and Lock 1987). Third, the majority of the authors working with this orientation would assume that medical knowledge includes certain ideas and beliefs that are "mystified" or "manipulated" by sections identified as more powerful. Nevertheless, one can never be sure if the apparently powerful position of biomedicine, for example, remains so all the way along and in all social and political/moral situations. Other differing systems may prove superior, though not purely from the perspective preferred by the dominant system. Health systems are cultural systems with their own worldviews. They have unique logic that may possess authority following the kind of problem or situation considered.

Ong's (1988) study of spirit possession in Sungai Jawa, a village (*Kampung*) based in the Kuala Langat district of Malaysia, offers a good example of the perspective brought by political economy studies. It also illustrates the theoretical approach I use in my study. The study begins by recognizing that possession in Malaysia traditionally happened to married women in phases of transition between different social roles (for example, around the time when they get married and when they give birth to their first child). Also, a conventional explanation of possession used to center around the notion of transgression: it struck women who crossed boundaries that set them apart from the domains occupied by men. The author observes that a major change has recently happened. Possession now happens to young unmarried women. She links this change to the transformation ensuing from industrialization initiated by the influx of multinational factories into the region. As these enterprises sought a cheaper labor force, they hired tens of thousands of women who, as a result, had to move across the boundaries of their communities to work in spaces conventionally perceived as a property of men. Subsequently, these nubile women started to experience spirit attacks in the form of violent episodes of rage on the factory floors. As such, these incidents mark a change in the classic definition of possession as well as in its early social function of self-control. The author thus maintains,

> Like other cultural forms, spirit possession incidents may acquire new meanings and speak to new experiences in changing arenas of social relations and boundary definitions . . . This transition from *Kampung* to urban industrial contexts has cast village girls into an intermediate status that they find unsettling and fraught with danger to themselves and to Malay culture (*ibid*: 32).

Parallel to this change in the definition of spirit possession, the discourse around the management of the affliction changed. Biomedical therapies such as doses of sedatives were used along with the ritualistic sessions of the *bomoh* (traditional healer) who was called up by the factory management to exorcise the factory area, which formerly was a graveyard believed to be inhabited by ancestral spirits.

Overall, Ong interprets possession as an intricate language of the body that expresses feelings of alienation from production, bodies and social relations in the factory (*ibid*: 34). This new combinatory management of the affliction maintained, if not intensified, the fear from spirit possession, which is interpreted by Ong as a means of resistance on the part of the workers. As a result, the methods of therapy created "self-regulation on the part of the workers" (*ibid*: 35).

Ong's paper provides an illustration for my theoretical orientation. It shows how "mixes" of therapies function to maintain the social order which is maintained and resisted by bodily language aired during sickness episodes and formulated with reference to social discourse that includes different, though interlinked, ideological frameworks that represent social and economic relationships characterized by friction and resistance.

POLITICS, ECONOMICS AND MORALITY IN HEALTH TERMS

E. P. Thomson suggests using the term *moral economy* as a field within which people from different social backgrounds hold beliefs that defend traditional rights or customs assumed to be supported by the wider consensus of the community. This assumption was occasionally affirmed by explicit support from central authorities operating within a popular consensus on the legitimacy of various economic practices regarding the making and distribution of food. This consensus was grounded within a historically rooted view of social norms defining "obligations, of the proper economic functions of several parties within the community, which, taken together, can be said to constitute the moral economy of the poor" (1971: 78–89). Thompson argues that this economy is ultimately political; it stems from "supposed definite, and passionately held, notions of the common weal" (*ibid*: 79). Furthermore, these notions are simultaneously employed within the tradition for purposes of power. In the context of eighteenth-century England Thompson notes that these notions "re-echoed so loudly in their turn that the authorities, in some measure, were the prisoners of the people" (*ibid*: 79).

In divided societies like Egypt life conditions, including those concerned with politics and the economy, are viewed and managed in diverse ways across different social groups. In contexts of plurality, a discourse must ensue between the groups concerned. This is the exact subject of this study; the way notions of life, wellness, health, illness, and death, and the values and forms of reasoning associated with them, are shared and unshared by focusing on what I call their morality. I suggest that this takes place through a moral discourse on social health.

Egypt has been directly colonized by western powers and then ruled by national elites who depended on foreign forces. More significantly, the entire country has been subject to massive modernizing projects that led to privileging European knowledge systems over local ones. Health care systems were included. In an insightful article, Peter Gran (1979a) argues that modern biomedical services prevailed because the Egyptian national bourgeoisie encouraged their spread and never tried to sustain or develop their inherited medical traditions. Gran's views are particularly instructive for studies of plurality. They certainly help avoid Eurocentric assumptions on non-European histories and thus open paths for further critical studies illustrating how apparently western socioeconomic and cultural phenomena such as capitalism and secularism may have occurred in other traditional contexts like eighteenth-century Egypt.[12] The question that interests me here is not whether traditional health practices have persisted, because there is ample evidence for their surviving and even flourishing.[13] More relevant is the way they have developed under different political economic arrangements and the kind of conceptual and institutional alignments they have engaged *in practice*. For example, has the biomedical separation between the body and the mind changed Egyptian cultural perceptions of life, or is that process of change part of a complex interaction between theoretical constructions and complex lived realities? Do the values upheld by different medical systems enjoy the same amounts of power in all contexts? Or there is somehow a "cultural logic" specific to the

Egyptian context that enables people to criticize various therapies based on different situations run according to local cultural logics? This last question is of special interest; I am interested in the diverse ways social relations are expressed in health and medicine-related terms and the implications of the resulting articulations for our understanding of health as a moral discourse—as a social practice undertaken by groups characterized by different ideological orientations.

Since the second half of the last century, Egypt has had a centrally run economy where the state owned and controlled the economy and spheres of life in health care, education, and law. It even developed its own version of Islamic teachings by co-opting, or rather buying off, reliable religious leaderships while oppressing others critical of its policies. That mode was called Nasserism, which included adapting to a socialist economy and lasted until the mid-1970s. During that period, the population slowly grew accustomed to the state taking care of their various needs. By the end of the 1960s paternalistic feelings were rampant; Nasser was literally and practically described as the father of the nascent nation that had just been liberated from the grip of traditional colonialism. The period this study focuses upon is the twenty-five years that followed. Egypt started to witness a particular socio-economic transformation associated with radical shifts toward a free market economy.

Much of the former state has survived but only formally; subsidized supplies and services, including those concerned with health care, remain but with a much lower quality. A five-minute tour in the main and oldest hospital in Cairo, al-Qasr al-Aini, traditionally an icon for the greatest two-hundred-year-old modernist enterprise, bears witness to the deterioration. Patients stay in huge wards. Their beds are barely covered with basic linens. Broken windows allow tens of sparrows to freely fly in and out. Patients have to contribute toward the cost of their treatment. Those who need surgery, for example, have to buy part of the paraphernalia required from the market.

In the mid-1990s, when I did the field research for this book, private enterprise was growing massively at the expense of a public sector presented in the media as inefficient and losing. That growth was associated with an increased sense of deterioration for the majority of the population. Starting with the mid-1980s, a piercing smell of corruption started to fill the air. Government officials were suspected of having entered the private sector; important public sector assets were repeatedly sold for much lower prices than their market value. The owners laid off laborers. Soon, it would become clear that state officials were major shareholders in the new companies buying up state assets. The public, used to a paternal sense toward the state, would feel betrayed. Those who benefited were so few. The number who grew poorer and poorer increased massively. A tense sense of division has already taken root in society (cf. Marfleet 2009: 28–31).[14]

These massive transformations were not always clearly defined by the subjects of this study. Particular circumstances in the immediate environment of the individuals, however, were assumed to be ultimately manifestations of something larger operating at the scale of society as a whole. Included, as we see in chapter 3, are crowdedness, pollution, soaring prices associated with a compromised sense of trust and compromised degree of morality, and excessive encroaching of materialist values in place of long-held beliefs and norms.

In this charged atmosphere, the general feeling was the continued deterioration in living standards that could not be explained by a lack of resources, but by defective ways of managing these and sharing them properly. It was suspected that something major had gone wrong or, in health-moral terms, become incorrect. It is *al-fasād* or corruption, which is a notion used to describe the economy, political power, and social integration. Simultaneously, it is a health-related concept applying to physical and mental conditions that have been irreversibly compromised. It also applies to the health of water and air, and relates to long-standing theories for explaining epidemics. It is actually an old theory. In all cases there is implied a lack of general balance or a feeling of injustice. Interestingly, this recalls a centuries-old theory that tried to explain general ill-health by the miasma: "the stench arising from swamps and putrefying organic matter, contained a toxic element that could vitiate the atmosphere and cause disease in susceptible individuals who were exposed to the noxious fumes." (Kuhnke 1990: 3). The moral implications of this theory relate to the fact that susceptible individuals are characterized by excessive indulgence. The miasmatic theory provided the logic upon which many health related reforms in the nineteenth-century England were based (*ibid*). I would further suggest that in the case of Egypt some meanings of this theory are still at work and they travel further to include the morality of life conditions in a much more comprehensive, and thus critical, fashion.

This book includes observations and detailed descriptive data gathered over eighteen months of fieldwork conducted in one old-standing neighborhood of Cairo. These data present the way life in the city and the country as a whole looks and *feels* through the eyes and minds of ordinary people living the city's worsening conditions. Interestingly, these views correspond with a nationwide discourse on the moral correctness of life in contemporary Egypt represented by major authors like Alaa al-Aswaani (2010), Galal Amin (1988), and Galal Aamer (2010).[15] A prominent example relevant to health issues is al-Aswani's *Why do the Egyptians not Revolt?* (*limātha lā yathūru al-misriyyūn*). Many others have also become mouthpieces for the feelings spread among the public. The author is a dentist, a novelist, and political activist. More recently he became a major figure in the revolution of 25 January 2011. In the aforementioned widely distributed book he lists many of the issues mentioned by the persons I met during field research, including the pressure of economic life, pollution, overcrowded cities, and the way low quality services are outer expressions for some serious issues that went seriously wrong. Further, the morals of society embodied by the central authorities have been exceedingly compromised and sickened the very social fabric.

These works are too many to be reviewed here. The reason I mention them in this introductory chapter is methodological; they point to the fact that many of the feelings and thoughts that occur and take root in the local environments are *discursively* connected to those circulated at the scale of society and national culture at large. What I am trying to say in this book is that the realities in which we live in a contemporary society are multilayered and too complex to be explained by reference to forces operating in local communities alone. The latter are ultimately creatures of discourses able to make and remake localities in new forms and content and following the changing, shifting, and uneven positions and links of power. This view made me study health practices in several "cultural sites" concerned with sustaining and improving life in direct and indirect ways including the family, the clinic, and the general public.

The question that arises here is the manner in which the life and health of individuals are mediated through all these complex levels. The answer that this book offers consists of the old-standing notion of *al-nafs* as a shared moral being able to host discourses on the life of living persons and not mere individuals, communities, and societies constructed in abstract terms. I believe that *al-nafs* derives its power from so many diverse threads shared in different proportions and manners by all members of society and concerned with defining what it means to be human.

This study draws observations from several sites relating to the central question of how the body, health, and wellness are subjectively experienced within the present socioeconomic conditions characterized by a prominent postcolonial state associated with a growing free market, increased sense of intense physical distress emanating from social and emotional adverse conditions. Chapter 1 explores the health resources available through an approach that highlights how these are culturally perceived and introduced by the practitioners who run them. Chapter 2 examines how persons experience different therapies in the context of family life. Chapter 3 focuses on a social epidemic called *'iḍḍaghṭ* that brings emotions and the explanatory power for understanding the role of subjectivity in connection to the notion of *al-nafs*. Chapter 4 illustrates that constructions of the body, life, wellness, illness, and death are never static. These are continually debated in ways illustrating various forms of conflict and cooperation occurring at the level of society at large. Chapter 5 moves further in society to examine how the body is constructed by authoritative institutions by relying on the various concepts and ideas provided by the plural system of wellness, not only of the individual but the entire society. Finally, Chapter 6 brings in some concluding remarks and questions for future research.

NOTES

1. The availability of therapies belonging to different traditions in single communities has been a salient feature of life in most populations of today's world. The literature on this theme is voluminous. There are, however, some seminal works that shaped this concept in when it was first developed in the early seventies of the twentieth century including Leslie, Charles (ed.), (1976), *Asian Medical Systems: A Comparative Study*. Berkeley: University of California Press; Young, Allan, and Charles Leslie *Paths to Asian Medical Knowledge*. Berkeley: University of California Press (1992); and Nichter, Mark, and Margaret Lock (2002), *New Horizons in Medical Anthropology: Essays in Honour of Charles Leslie*. London: Routledge.
2. For a fuller account about the *Mulids* of *Būlāq*, see Gilsenan (1973: 47–64).
3. To mention but a few the book of Abu Hamid al-Ghazaali, the eleventh-century scholar, and *ihyā 'ulūm al-dīn* (Revival of Religious Sciences), see www.ghazali.org/ihya/ihya.htm for a full website dedicated to this magnum opus. Dr. Mohammed Qutb on the other hand is a contemporary scholar who works to maintain and develop al-Ghazali's work on *al-nafs*. See Mohammed Qutb (2005), *dirasāt fi al-nafs al-'insāniyyah* (Studies of the human soul). Al-Qahira: Dar al-Shurooq.
4. Modern biomedicine itself has been subject to critical anthropological studies for many years now. This book however is not directly related to this subject which has been variously investigated by Good and Good (1993); Good and Good (1993); Latour and Woolgar (1986); Rapp (1993); Traweek (1993).
5. There are innumerable studies on these issues. Most, however, rely on utilitarian models of therapeutic action, as noted by Comaroff (1980: 638). They perceive individuals as autonomous and rational agents rather than actors bound to historically produced social structures. It seems that the trend to focus on traditional healing to include them in official medical systems started before the Al-maata conference. Examples include Frankenberg (1973) in a sociological paper on Zambia, Zaire, and China. For later periods, see Heggenhougen (1987) for Malaysia.
6. Underlying Janzen's words are important distinctions and assumptions. First and foremost is the distinction between the "western" and the "non-western." The western is seen as modern, physical, tangible, real, and so forth. The non-western is nonmodern. Implied is that it is mystical, less tangible, social, religion-based, and so forth. These distinctions have long been criticized by anthropologists such as Marcus and Fisher (1986), Csordas and Kleinman (1990), and Good (1995), as will be discussed subsequently.

7. Many anthropologists describe the way different therapies are perceived by people keep "as" complementary, and conflictual relationships (see McCormack 1981 for example). These attempts, however, lead nowhere near deciding on a single and unchanging relationship. As Lewis and Frankel (1989) suggest, the ways people accept or reject different therapies are complex and highly varied and thus "difficult to place . . . all under the head of one or two general processes, or one or two common attitudes. What might one take? Integration? Opposition? A pragmatism that is materialist and realist? Empirical curiosity? Closed conservatism? Millenarian enthusiasm? Magical outlook? Syncretic openness? Opportunism? Political pressure? Distribution of resources and access to them? Beliefs about power? Eagerness for modern things, progress and 'cargo'? Differences of education and information? Shrewd assessment on the basis of limited evidence? Religious persuasion? Charismatic and forceful leaders? Innocence or ignorance?" (*ibid*: 25).

8. When looked at from the perspective of embodiment and experience, the processes of interaction between different therapeutic methods produce complex configurations of practice. The metaphor of "latticed knowledge" that Parkin (1995) uses to describe the minute interweaving dynamics of medical knowledge in contemporary Muslim society applies here strongly.

9. These studies are inspired and guided in various degrees by the theory of the world capitalist system. This literature is too voluminous to review here. See Wallerstein (1974) for the general theoretical paradigm, Rodney (1974) for the case of Africa, and Amin (1989) for the notion of eurocentrism associated with the rise, development, and expansion of Europe as a colonial power in both economic and cultural terms. Nash (1981) provides a good overview of the development and use of these theoretical works in anthropology.

10. For a systematic introduction of the spatial, causal, and time connections between the micro and macro levels of analysis see DeWalt and Pelto (1985: 1–21, 187–200).

11. Some of the proponents of the political economy of health suggest using the expression "critical medical anthropology" (see Singer 1990) for their approach. I think this label is misleading and has little significance when comparing between different theoretical approaches. It is misleading because any process of seeking knowledge, which is one of the tasks of medical anthropology, is *critical* by definition. The word "critical" is related to the word "crisis." Both share the same Latin root (see Koselleck 1988: fn.103–104). The relationship between the two words is, of course, far more complex than this simple relationship. However, it is enough to indicate one problem with the current use of the term "critical." There is no doubt that much medical anthropology, including that criticized by the so-called "critical medical anthropologists," has been written in response to a crisis felt in the modern medical care services (see Csordas and Kleinman 1990, or an even older essay by Kleinman, Eisenberg, and Good 1978).

12. See, for example, Peter Gran (1979a), *Islamic Roots of Capitalism: 1760–1840*. Austin: University of Texas Press for a history of eighteenth-century Egypt illustrating the development of capitalist relations of production well before the invasion of European powers. Some of these studies go too far in considering modern biomedicine as a science reproduced in highly regulated environments (Strathern

1992). I think it is not necessary or sensible to define science in rigid parameters. In fact, much of the medical practice takes place in clinics, hospitals, drugstores, and even homes. In all cases these are the spaces that concern me.

13. See, for example, Inhorn (1996), Morsy (1978), and Lane and Millar (1987). I will also discuss how these therapies still survive in texts continuously produced for self-help (see chapter 2).

14. The volume edited by Mahdi and Marfleet provides an excellent overview of the developments that occurred in the period of my study and which led to major social, economic, and political transformations.

15. These books are originally collections of articles written by the authors over long periods and published in many local newspapers. They must have reached millions of readers. Likewise, the books too have been reprinted many times; for instance, al-Aswani's books that have been reprinted no less than twenty times each.

1

Healing Contemporary Life

Examples of Popular Self-Help Guides

In this chapter I explore popular self-help guides written by health practitioners. I argue that these guides demonstrate that contemporary Egyptian health practices constitute a plural system organized around local cultural principles and ideals represented primarily by Islam. The relationship between different resources is sometimes conflictual. However, it is operated in creative ways leading to a synthesis of composite forms of therapy responsive to the dilemmas of contemporary society while rooted in cultural memory. The new forms are marked by a quest for holism; they bring together elements from the law, religion, and both Prophetic and modern medicine to tackle emerging social and health problems. Health in this context corresponds perfectly to the notion of *al-ṣiḥḥah,* interpreted at the beginning of the last chapter to mean correctness or justice. This understanding of health views physical well-being as a result of an optimum balance connecting different elements of life that enmesh the body within a constellation of immaterial concepts that include the soul, the spirit, the mind, society, emotions, and so forth. These concepts and the way they are constructed and related to each other, of course, vary from one author to another. Nevertheless, all authors insist that they are essential for a proper understanding of health. Second, most of these pamphlets recognize that modern biomedicine is very useful and necessary. However, it is insufficient because it covers mere materials aspects of life. Their plurality, therefore, aims at crossing borders between systems of medical care so that while maintaining and or restoring health they would also preserve the sense of dignity and integrity of human life. Therefore, the authors explicitly call for resistance against the use of modern biomedicine including its assumptions about life and society. It is most interesting that these pamphlets confirm the observation that the concepts of disease or illness are essentially different.

They certainly overlap but their respective meanings are independent of each other. The former is bodily while the latter is related to beliefs and concepts shared by both patients and healers. Finally, most of these pamphlets aim at escaping rigid material definitions of biomedicine in order to accommodate moral and religious meanings into health and healing. The exception is one pamphlet trying to appropriate the traditional concept of *al-nafs* to realize further control and surveillance over individuals: this will be clear toward the end of the chapter.

MEDICAL PLURALISM IN COMPARATIVE PERSPECTIVE

Nicholas Rose's (2006) study on biopolitics of life in the contemporary world society provides a useful backdrop to discuss the materials of this chapter. He notes that conflicting views and desires surround the late biomedical inventions. A drive toward profit is faced by morality contestations engaged by healers, philosophers, intellectuals, scientists, and ethicists among others. The issues debated link medical practices to society and social norms in direct and indirect ways. Rose is not concerned with taking sides in these debates. He is focused on analyzing speculations and meditations as visions of the future that include fears and hopes, evaluations and judgments as elements of emerging forms of life burgeoning in the context of changing medical technologies. Rose's work however is only partly relevant to my interest in medical pluralism. He declares that he is mainly concerned with the "growing capacities of medical technologies to control, manage, engineer, reshape, and modulate the very vital capacities of human beings as living creatures." In a word, he is concerned with the politics of *life itself*. It becomes directly relevant when he notes that the current modifications in rationalities technologies have been associated with increased desires of individuals to take responsibility for their life by managing self-styled activities to gain further security toward the future. His analysis too concerns developments in advanced liberal democracies including complex of "marketization, autonomization, and responsibilization" (Rose 2006: 3–4).

Rose rightly argues that the reshaping of medical and political perception and practice has been taking place along the following dimensions: (1) *Molecularization* or excessive emphasis on molecular forms of life that are isolated and manipulated in the laboratory. But this category is far from being relevant to the Egyptian situation. Biotechnologies are not that sophisticated in Egypt. (2) *Optimization*, which refers to seeking the best possibilities of the available health care resources. I believe this is very comparable to the Egyptian situation although for particular reasons connected to the traditional understanding of health as an optimum state of being as discussed in the introduction. (3) *Subjectification* or the drive toward conceptualizing human life in pure biological forms and taking these as final reference of what life should and could be is too different because it is inserted within a different cultural milieu. In particular, the health pamphlets included in this chapter place immense amount of significance on the notion of *al-nafs*, which is an uncertain field that does not draw complete lines between active and passive forms of being. As such, it gives a great amount of autonomy, or this is at least what the desire is, for deciding various meanings of various issues of life, health and well-being, and death. In addition, *al-nafs* as will be discussed in the final chapter on organ donation is of practical value in this world; it points to an immortal capacity that continues to have significance after death. (4) *Somatic expertise*, which means that these techniques led by geneticists, cell therapists, and other highly specialized experts ultimately assist in governing human conduct that contributes to humans controlling human behavior. This argument that in present society we have been witnessing the rise of "somatic individuals" linked to the development of "somatic ethics" sharply contrasts with the practice examined in this chapter. I would argue that in Egypt the drive may be going to the opposite direction. Most of the pamphlets presented here are calling for shifting the emphasis off the body to *al-nafs* as an holistic capacity presenting human life in its entirety. (5) *Economies of vitality* motivated by the search for biovalue: the issue of capitalization, the demands for shareholder value, and the human value invested in the hope for cure and optimality. This is generally a possibility for the case of Egypt and the reason is the rapid growth of the market economy that has certainly impacted investments in medical care. But in the particular case of the pamphlets I think they have possibly grown because of the very growth of the market to provide self-help that may be accessible and affordable and thus provides a sense of autonomy from the market.

A NOTE ON METHODS

Methods to analyze texts include hermeneutics, narrative and discourse analysis, schema analysis grounded theory, and content analysis (Bernard 2006: x). This chapter is concerned with the last two methods, which are very widely used in social sciences today. Grounded theory is concerned with the discovery and labeling of concepts (variables) and the building of models based on a close reading of the text. It aims at building a hypothesis based on surveyed concepts. Content analysis is centered on the formal description of concepts and the testing of models and hypotheses (Bernard 2006: 492).

This chapter dwells on ethnographic materials based on a well-confirmed observation that the health care system in Egypt is plural. No need is there to further prove this fact and thus grounded theory is not particularly relevant. Likewise, content analysis starts with a hypothesis before coding the material. That is its deductive part. The idea is to test whether the hypothesis involved is correct. Next, it seeks to inductively explore and discover the way different facts are operating in particular contexts (Bernard 2006: 493).

A complete content analysis should include a group of texts, a theory to test, a set of codes for variables to measure reliability that assists in creating a unit-of-analysis-by-variable matrix. Finally, the matrix is analyzed statistically (Bernard 2006: 507). The content analysis I am conducting in this chapter is not that methodologically complex. It aims at presenting an underexplored ethnographic site ensuing from the plural nature of the health system in Egypt: the ever proliferating texts authored by diverse medical practitioners searching for solutions for emerging health concerns. My aim is to highlight major concepts deployed in this field and aiming at moral-political ends rather than purely therapeutic ones. The aim too is to discuss the regulatory concepts that permeate other ethnographic sites investigated in the other chapters. My arguments is that these concepts ultimately reflect how subjectivity is shaped within the modern space of printed texts.

KEEPING WELL IN MODERN SOCIETY: A GENERAL OVERVIEW

Various professional, economic, and therapeutic interests underlie the publication of these pamphlets. It is important to remember that health practitioners pursue these interests in an environment marked by multiple physical and ecological problems that bear direct relevance to contemporary, economic, and political conditions. Practitioners are aware of these problems. Many authors view these problems as products of what they call "modern life." The assumption is that modern society in Egypt has health problems unique to modern life. Simultaneously, available health resources became inadequate. Many authors view existing therapies, including biomedicine, as inherently insufficient to deal with important dimensions of health care. In this context, the authors of pamphlets reformulate both existing and new therapies in ways assumed to enhance their efficacy. However, the issue is not purely practical, I would firmly argue; the concepts of the body and the soul and the way they are interwoven are deeply rooted in Egyptian history. They describe not only individual health and illness, but also the health of society at large. This is simply the way health has been constructed traditionally. My argument is that the process of reformulating therapies provides practitioners with a medium to disseminate social, religious, and political messages along with their therapeutics. By medium I mean the complex amalgam of ideas and therapies synthesized from different sources. The significant issue here is the plurality that helps produce coherent articulations compatible with the society's traditional values regarding health care and its role in enforcing social order.

The plural character of Egyptian medical and health practices has been discussed and documented by anthropologists and historians. Numerous scholars suggest that practices combine elements traceable to Pharaonic medicine, Yunani Greek medicine, Prophetic medicine and biomedicine. Certain studies focus on the historical origins of these practices (Bürgel 1976), and their general course of transformation (Gran 1976). Other studies investigate the continuation of practices from the past to the present (Millar and Lane 1988; al-Gammal n.d.). Many studies emphasize that health resources in Egypt are hierarchically organized and thus are not equitably distributed and available for different classes and genders (Lane and Millar 1987; Morsy 1980). In this chapter about pamphlets, I explore the following questions: what are the major sources of theorization about health and illness? How are the concepts that are commonly used to describe human well-being defined and used, including concepts of health, illness, body, soul, and mind? What circumstances are considered threats to health? Which forces are considered sources of healing? It is evident that the healers have coherent ideas and effective therapies based on a variety of sources. However, what best describes practitioners' processes of evaluating different methods of healing in different situations of *practice*? Can these be described as pragmatic, eclectic, syncretic, critical, flexible, or dogmatic? Finally, how do health practitioners view individual health in relation to the health of society?

First, I present an overview of the pamphlets. Then, I focus on pamphlets which explicitly discuss concepts of the body, health and illness, and which I assume represent medical traditions at work in contemporary society. In particular, I discuss the concept of "modern life" as used by different authors. I focus on concepts of health (*al-ṣiḥḥah*) and illness (*al-maraḍ*) in connection with concepts of the body (*al-jasad*), the soul (*al-nafs*), the spirit (*al-rūḥ*), the mind (*al-'aql*), and the heart (*al-qalb*). Finally, I discuss different therapies recommended in the pamphlets. I focus on the principles used in deciding on therapies rather than on therapies themselves. I conclude with a summary that links the results of this chapter to the rest of the book.

WHAT ARE THE PAMPHLETS?

The pamphlets included are booklets similar in size and shape. They consist of 100 to 150 pages with colorful drawings on their covers. Many covers show human organs or the whole body, sometimes surrounded by assorted herb collections or medical instruments. Sold in Cairo's bookshops, at newspaper kiosks, or by sidewalk vendors, these booklets are widely available. Their prices vary from three to seven Egyptian pounds, affordable to many people from middle-income groups.

The average pamphlet consists of a brief introduction (one to three pages) followed by a therapeutic section that contains the illnesses and problems with which the pamphlet deals. At the end is a list of references. Supporters of the author's ideas and therapies write introductions to some pamphlets. The therapeutic section is generally the most extensive. It includes diverse diseases and therapies. Reference sections in most of the pamphlets frequently list books used by the author but they are not cited in the text. It is difficult to know which ideas are the author's own. It is possible only to guess this when the style of sentences changes because the references used are mostly in classical Arabic. The authors, however, are not concerned with making that difference clearer by giving the sources for other texts. The reason might be that quotations from older texts are already known well enough for readers to be aware that they belong to different sources. Another possibility is that the authors are attempting to imply that their texts are continuations of older texts. There is no doubt that authors would benefit from the authority implied by older texts.

The pamphlets demonstrate that understandings of health and illness are neither homogeneous nor free from outside influences. Authors rework different ideas for various therapeutic, social, and political purposes. Some authors claim that they are aiming at improving the efficacy of the methods. Others claim that they interpret therapeutic methods into locally comprehensible terms. In many cases, medical ideas are deliberately integrated with social and religious rules and instructions. These rules and instructions have less to do with what we may *analytically* identify as physical well-being than with social well-being, as envisaged by health practitioners concerned with the integrity of a larger social order. Clearly, the relative position of different ideas must be subject to change depending on varying circumstances and situations as mentioned above. I am however particularly concerned with how concepts originating in medicine are simultaneously integrated in larger frameworks that ultimately influence social and political relations.

As noted above, the majority of the pamphlets provide information and therapies for specific physical problems and complaints. These pamphlets are the most widely available. They discuss commonly known ailments such as high blood pressure, kidney problems, back pain, and sexual and reproductive problems. Most pamphlets contain biochemical and herb therapies. Some pamphlets introduce healing methods primarily based on the notion of faith (*'imān*). Their authors claim that their treatments are only based on the Quran and the Prophet's tradition. Such pamphlets are part of a religious-social movement known as the Islamic revival. Some authors include official letters from the government religious authority of al-Azhar University approving their methods and attesting that their therapies do not contradict the rules of *al-Shari'a* (Islamic jurisprudence). In addition, there are pamphlets that introduce methods of treating illnesses caused by sorcery and magic. Other pamphlets contain no specific therapeutic methods. They consist of reflections on the current landscape of health and illness. These are concerned with social rather than individual illnesses. They are about conditions, circumstances, and practices that promote health or engender illness in society, whether directly or indirectly.

The authors who write and publish these pamphlets are diverse. Most display knowledge in more than one field of expertise. Some cover medical, religious, social, and political issues. The pamphlets are good examples of the way medical knowledge is transformed in its interaction with society and culture. Authors include physicians, sheikhs, psychiatrists, herb therapists, and persons specializing in physical therapy. The influence of the authors' cultural backgrounds is evident in their writings: physicians studied at the medical school of al-Azhar University and draw upon the religious concepts and healing methods of this institution. Al-Azhar has been the source of myriad manuscripts written by Muslim scholars and physicians throughout the past several hundred years. Quranic healers also studied at al-Azhar. Next to physicians, there are therapists who call themselves herb experts (*'ashshābīn* or *'aṭṭārīn*). These therapists introduce their medicines by using terms from biomedicine and other theories of treatment such as the humoral theory. An example is one pamphlet written by the proprietor of an herb shop (al-Harraaz 1994). This pamphlet is an example of how practitioners tend to synthesize new therapies as composite forms that are more relevant to what is identified as the sickness or problem at hand. The use of biomedical terms shows an awareness of a conflict in authority between biomedicine and other forms of medicine and by drawing on them they are proposing *de facto* a synthesis between them. In his introduction, al-Harraaz (1994) addresses physicians and other scientists by saying: "go back to our heritage . . . where laboratory tests can be combined with what popular medicine has achieved through experiments and observation" (*ibid*: 9). Another example is a pamphlet entitled "Magical Prescriptions of Medicinal Herbs" (*waṣfāt jinnyah li al-'ilāg bi al-'a'shāb al-ṭibbiyyah*) by Mohammed Abduh Maghawri (1995). This author uses past medical works such as *Tathkirat Dā'ūd* by Daa'ud bin Omar al-Antaaki, Prophetic Medicine by Ibn al-Qayyim, *al-qānūn fi al-ṭib* by Ibn Sina (Avicena), all of which are widely recognized as standard references for Islamic medicine. This pamphlet shows the way traditional medical knowledge based on humoral theory accommodates recently emerging disease categories. The author explains that high blood pressure results from increased electrical charges in the brain. Therefore it belongs to the hot-dry diseases that should be treated with moist therapies (*ibid*: 37).

MODERN LIFE AND ILLNESS

Many authors use the concept of "modern life" to explain the reasons behind publishing their pamphlets, or point to factors that engender disease in contemporary society. Most authors indicate ambivalence about aspects of modern society, especially with regard to modern biomedicine. On the one hand, they show great appreciation of various advances in modern science. On the other hand, the same authors are critical of phenomena associated with recent urbanization and industrialization. In the introduction' to "Diseases of the Present Time between Science and Religion" (*'amrād al'aṣr bayna al-'ilm wa al-dīn*), Al-Gamal (1993) states: "I want to analyze problems of my time which emerged in midst of modern civilizations, and which have been produced by great changes and scientific inventions" (*ibid*: 5). He lists many problems of modern life; most importantly, what he calls "sickness of the soul" (*ibid*: 73). In a statement that defines what might be called feelings of dissonance, he explains that sickness of the soul means "irregularity in ideas, lack of stability, and inconsistency in people's actions" (*ibid*). While this is very abstract, in the present context it is enough to indicate that "modern life" is an ethnographic category used by many authors. They argue that contemporary society has many disease-engendering conditions. The endemic spread of diabetes, for instance, is ascribed to "the modern life style" which is characterized by too much bodily rest or inertia, and tension (al-Hussaini 1994b: 15). In such a condition, "many of our diseases persisted despite the great progress achieved by humanity" (al-Hussaini 1994a: 6–7). Al-Hussaini adds that "our conventional chemical therapies are unable to correct damage caused by diseases, and if they do, they produce many undesirable side effects" (*ibid*). The aim of rethinking biochemical therapies goes beyond repairing specific physical problems produced by this form of treatment. In fact, modern biomedicine here is viewed as inseparable from modern ways of life springing from the expansion of the market noted early on in the last chapter. This observation lends support to my argument that health care views are reformulated to form a cultural critique not merely of physical problems but of society as a whole and its recent transformations.

RETHINKING MODERN BIOMEDICINE

Some practitioners introduce therapies with a call to rethink modern biomedicine. In "Seven Doctors from Nature: Treatment without Surgery or Drugs" (*Sab' 'ṭibā' min al-ṭabī'ah: al-'ilāg bidūn girāḥah aw dawlā'*), Mohammed Kamaal Abdel'aziz (1992) focuses on a call to "seek therapy and healing by natural" materials. He contrasts the "natural" with the synthetic therapies. Nevertheless, he emphasizes that he is not calling people "to turn or look backward or to repudiate scientific achievements." His call is to use "natural means of therapy in connection with the startling progress achieved by laboratory experiments and research" (*ibid*: 5). His call is to employ scientific knowledge by placing it in a framework that gives primacy to "nature." But what does he mean by nature? A closer look at the way the author uses this category reveals that the difference between the "natural" and whatever might stand in opposition is rather complicated. His distinction is an abstract construction. In the eyes of Abdel'aziz, nature represents what remains free from human "manufacturing and distortion," and thus still retains "the original elements that the great God has placed in them" (*ibid*: 7). The distinction then is between two spaces of living, so to speak, one divinely given and the other humanly created. The first is original, pure and beneficial; the second is transformed, temporary and unsafe or even harmful. I argue that this idea lends support to my earlier definition of health as a state of correctness and integrity. Health then is an aspiration toward originality and purity, which I think are presented as a critique of the current culture implicitly assumed to be artificial and contaminated. Such culture is most probably the current way of life in Cairo associated with the expansion of the market economy, industrialization, and consumerism as is clear below.

How did humans turn out to be polluting? The author asserts that humans polluted the environment with toxic materials, including the air and medicines that also contain great amounts of toxic materials (*ibid*: 6). Food is polluted because it contains preservatives. Moreover, "present mechanical life makes people eat quickly and eat processed foods" (*ibid*). These issues, Abdel'aziz continues, mark the "deep abyss into which this ceaseless rhythm of modern life has thrown us" (*ibid*: 8). Subsequently he calls for a new medical system based on a "return to nature" and focused on the "body's self-repairing powers." Finally, the author maintains that everything artificial needs to be avoided. Artificiality is disease engendering, according to his perspective. He calls for a rethink of biochemical drugs in order to maintain health by the use of natural materials represented by water, air, the sun, and other gifts from God. Abdel'aziz insists that people who take unhealthy materials often develop emotions of anger, fear, and anxiety. These are aggravated by adverse social and economic conditions. Such emotions impede the process of waste disposal and are responsible for illnesses such as high blood pressure, asthma, anemia, rheumatoid arthritis, and ulcers. Abdel'aziz's perspective views illness as originating not only in emotional and physical conditions but also in the surrounding material conditions.

Abdel'aziz's call to return to nature includes therapies which he says have roots in ancient Pharaonic, Chinese, Indian, and Babylonian medical traditions. He maintains that these "natural" therapies treat the patient as one comprehensive unit. The natural is a construction of the past where a pure, healthy state of being is imagined. This imaginary past should be revived to overcome contemporary illnesses. Other therapists follow similar reasoning in their pamphlets (Fahmi n.d.; al-Gammaal n.d.; Mukhtaar 1993; Shalabi 1995a, 1995b, 1995c). They underscore the pragmatic quest for therapy. Abdel'aziz is among the very few who explain the moral and social dimensions of his therapies for the illnesses he addresses.

MODERN MEDICINE AND THE QURAN

One pamphlet is entitled *The Inimitability of the Quranic Meanings of the Human Senses: A Study in the Ear, the Nose and the Larynx in Light of the Quranic Sciences and the Prophetic Tradition* (*'i'jāz al-qur'ān fi hawās al-'insān: dirāsah fi al-'anf wa al-'uthun wa al-ḥunjarah fi ḍuu' al-ṭib wa 'ulūm al-qur'ān wa al-hadith*). The author is physician Mohammed Kamaal Abdel'aziz, from al-Azhar University (1987). The introduction to this pamphlet was written by a senior professor from the same university. This professor notes that the pamphlet is "a scent of modern science blended with the breath of faith extending from the author's heart" (*ibid*: 8). It is interesting to examine how science is blended with religion and the messages implicit in this way of introducing religion in a medical scientific idiom. The author discusses the medical and theological meanings of the nose, the ear, and the larynx. In three sections, each devoted to one of the three organs, he explains the physiology and religious significance of these organs' functions: smell, hearing, and speaking. He is concerned with the metaphysical meanings of these functions as mentioned in the Quran. Abdel'aziz argues that medicine is insufficient to interpret these functions. According to him, God has endowed different individuals with different powers in different senses. Some individuals are only able to communicate with their physical and direct social surroundings. Others are granted stronger powers to receive divine messages, such as those possessed by the Prophet. The Prophet's companions and other devout believers are endowed with such powers based on their piety. Powerful senses thus can be developed through observing religious duties, which brings people closer to God. Rulers should be selected from those who are closer to God. This author evokes both religious and medical power to seek pure political ends that have to do more with the social order than the physical body.

Medicine in the Quran and the Prophet's Tradition (*al-ṭib fi al-qurān wa al-sunna: bayna al-dā 'wa al-dawā'*) by Mohammed Mahmoud Abdallah is a pamphlet illustrating continuing Islamic methods for conceptualizing health. Abdallah is a teacher of Quranic sciences at al-Azhar University. In the introduction, a physician working in the same university describes this book as a work that covers "medical and health benefits in the Quran because it combines the physical and spiritual aspects of human life" (*ibid*: 2). This pamphlet focuses on the concept of the heart (*al-qalb*). In contrast to illnesses of the heart that represent immaterial aspects of health, the author mentions illnesses of *al-badan* (the trunk). Illnesses of the heart include doubt (*shak*), excessive desire (*shahwa*), and hatred (*ghill*). Connected to this latter kind is a third group of pathological states that the author calls *al-'amrad al-nafsiyya* (illnesses of the soul). For the author, these illnesses result from emotional factors originating in public life such as fear (*al-khawf*), grief (*al-huzzn*), and fatigue (*al-ighaad*) (*ibid*: 8).

All psychological afflictions are related to the heart. But what is the heart? It is certainly not the biological organ. The author's awareness of the physical heart is assimilated within a larger understanding that he calls "the anatomical character of the heart in the Quran" (*ibid*: 9). Here, the heart is understood as a complex physical, perceptive, mental, intellectual, emotional, and spiritual entity. The general physiological functions of the heart are put in poetic-religious terms that view it as "the spring of life."

Abdallah's depiction of the heart encompasses five spaces. The first is *al-fu'aad*, which refers to the function of perception. It recognizes the apparent, which is a process of "ordinary understanding" (*ibid*: 11). Further, there is *al-lubaab*, which understands extraordinary, subtle, and hidden matters. It is not present in all individuals. Those who have stronger memories and can distinguish between the good and the bad attain it (*ibid*: 12). Within *al-lubaab* there exists *al-'aql* (the mind). *Al-'aql*'s functions are comparison, distinction, and reasoning. The heart and the mind are merged in the words of the author as he quotes the Quran in which reasoning is a function of the heart. Abdallah assumes that there should be no contradiction between the Quran and biomedicine. Inside *al-'aql* there is a fourth space called *al-wigdan* which is responsible for emotions. The final and most deeply located core of the heart is named *al-ginaan*, which holds the innermost, truthful beliefs that guide all human actions. For Abdallah, *al-ginaan* is the center where the name of God is recited by every beat. Further, it is where *al-yaqin* (absolute knowledge) is seated. Abdallah does not pursue elaborate methods of therapy based on his understanding of health. He simply lists some therapies along with illnesses. The social and political assumptions of Abdallah's therapies are not made explicit. Although not explicitly stated, Abdullah's description is somehow related to al-Ghazali's description of *al-nafs* mentioned in the last chapter. Whatever the case may be, the above construction of the heart places the greatest amount of emphasis on the integraptive roles emotions may play. This idea provides further support to the main thesis of this book, which will be focused upon in the last chapter.

A Guide for Therapists who Use the Quran (*dalil al-mu'ālijīn bil-qur'ān al-karīm*) by Mohammed Samaaha (1996) takes up the quest of formulating appropriate therapies. The pamphlet introduces definitions of body, soul, illness, health, and therapy in the context of what the author calls Quranic therapy. The latter refers to methods that rely on combining Quranic recitation but also include herbal remedies. Samaaha provides definitions of illnesses caused by spirit possession (*mas shaytāni*), magic (*siḥr*), and the evil eye (*ḥasad*). Then he provides a list of physical ailments together with their appropriate therapies. As references Samaaha lists the Quran and twenty-seven books authored by contemporary and past physicians and theologians. He also provides almost one hundred pages of newspapers clippings. These are commentaries, interviews, and reports written about himself and his work.

The author states that he is publishing his pamphlet because "illnesses and afflictions have spread around, and physicians have failed to cure patients who have been wandering around searching for an unattainable cure" (*ibid*: 7). The reason for these illnesses and afflictions is related to biomedicine, and perhaps to its general tendency to address illnesses as physical malfunctions separate from the culture in which they have been produced. Samaaha's pamphlet can be summarized by a statement in the introduction, which reads: "The living organs' quest [for healing] does not contradict the heart's certain knowledge (*al-yaqin*)" (*ibid*: 13). *Al-yaqin* is a religious philosophical concept that defines a complex mixture of knowledge and passion. *Al-yaqin* is the certitude of believing Muslims about their lives, the cause of their illnesses, and their fate. The statement connects sickness to processes of seeking help. In this context, sickness should be defined in terms of the knowledge that patients have about themselves. The body for Samaaha is mere material that "includes organs with spiritual meanings imperceptible for physical senses" (*ibid*: 10). The body is taken as a lived experience and not merely a physical entity. It is lived through five other capacities. These are the mind (*al-'aql*), the heart (*al-qalb*), the soul (*al-nafs*), the spirit (*al-rūh*), and the self (*al-thāt*) (*ibid*: 10–11). The author does not define these notions explicitly. He briefly notes that the mind represents abstract human thought and will, which are ultimately linked to God's will. The heart represents emotions; the soul has been formed by God; and the spirit is part of God's spirit. All these capacities are parts of the self. He quotes the Quran to imply that human knowledge is too limited to encompass these complex notions (*ibid*: 10). The meanings of these complex notions, however, appear through the way they are used in the rest of the pamphlet. Of the five concepts, only two are relevant to Samaaha's work: the mind and the spirit.

To define his field of expertise the author places the spirit in contrast with the body. His concern is with spiritual illnesses (*al-'amrāḍ al-rūḥiyya*) as opposed to physical ones (*al-'amrāḍ al-'ūḍwiyya*) (*ibid*: 11–13). To define notions of health and illness the author argues that the mind is the force that restores health, which takes place when the sick person restores his or her will over their body. The human body detached from these faculties is not part of the sheikh's field of expertise. In a note that defines what can be called a division of labor between the sheikh's field and that of physicians, he says that the body and its diseases are the focus of "human medicine" (*al-ṭib al-bashari*), which treats pure physical problems (*al-'amrāḍ al-'ūdwiyya al-baḥta*). Human medicine, he proceeds, is a necessary but insufficient means to realize and maintain good health. Treatment of all illnesses needs to include prayers for "God and in the words of God" (*ibid*: 11). Prayers are part of a consistent effort to maintain health and overcome illness. Next to pure bodily illness, Samaaha defines three other categories, including physical-spiritual illness (*maraḍ 'uḍwi rūḥi*), spiritual-physical illness (*maraḍ rūḥi 'uḍwi*), and purely spiritual illness (*maraḍ 'uḍwi baḥt*). This scheme is only practical. All illnesses have spiritual as well as material aspects. Identifying the kind of illness is helpful only in arranging priorities and steps of therapy (*ibid*: 13).

The sheikh lists complaints that he can assist people to overcome. Some of these are illustrated on the front cover of the pamphlet. They include *ṣudā'* (headache), *'ikti'āb* (depression), *waswās* (best translated as devilish, fixed, disquieting ideas), *nisyān* (forgetfulness), and *al-ṣudūd 'an al-tā'āt* (disobedience). These categories refer to symptoms rather than physical malfunctions. Samaaha is not concerned with the physical malfunctions that might underlie these symptoms. In medical anthropology the category of disease has been used in contrast to the categories of illness and sickness (see for example Frankenberg 1980; Young 1982). Disease is seen as defined by biomedicine. Illness refers to individuals' perception and experience of their physical discomfort. Sickness refers to the cultural and social definition of the former two categories. Samaaha's notion of unhealthy conditions is different. According to the implications of the above statement, categories of disease, illness, and sickness are merged and defined in terms shared between the healer and the help-seeker.

What terms does Samaaha use to indicate unhealthy conditions? He uses the term *marad*, which is the most widespread term in written Arabic in Egypt today. It is also used in everyday language in Cairo. It literally means corruption that results in any kind of weakness.[1]

Interestingly, it is used far beyond the context of individual cases of sickness to describe social pathologies so to speak, as will be seen later in this study. Colloquial Egyptian uses this term, together with another one called *'aya*, which means the person concerned is suffering from a state of weakness or tiredness. It is important to note here that in Egyptian Arabic there are other words to point to unhealthy conditions. These include *dā'* or *maraḍ*, and *'illa*. The first is concerned with processes of seeking therapy. In theory, for each *daa'* there should be a *dawaa'* (therapy). This idea is expressed by the common saying: *li-kulli daa'in dawaa'*. This saying is usually ascribed to the Prophet. The authors of many pamphlets also cite it. The term *dā'* is rarely used in everyday life away from this rhetorical context. The second term of *'illa* has a health-related meaning but is rarely used in spoken forms of Egyptian Arabic. But it is certainly used in poetry, songs, philosophy, and folk tales. The latter observation *further* illustrates how health-related ideas encompass different fields of life.

Samaaha's method for deciding that a person is *marīḍ* (sick) is symptomatologic. He suggests that spiritual afflictions (*'iṣābāt rūḥiyyah*) take place in moments of excessive anger, fear, sadness, or inattentiveness, meaning when the person is not observing their religious duties. Symptoms appear whether the person is awake or asleep. A person might have difficulty falling asleep, or have nightmares where they see snakes, spiders, dogs, cats, or other animals. Some speak while asleep, grind their teeth, walk, laugh, cry, or scream. They might feel they are falling from high places, or walk in graveyards. Upon awakening, people with spiritual afflictions might have headaches, increased pulse rate without doing additional effort, thoughts of murder or adultery, or excessive and involuntary rage. Some might have feelings of depression (*'ikti'āb*). These symptoms cannot be subsumed under one physical category. However, this is not Samaaha's concern. It is enough to see these symptoms to recognize spiritual illness. The sheikh states how he decides whether Satan harms the person,

> If all or some of the above symptoms are repeatedly noticed and they are strongly present . . . and make the person behave dramatically differently from before, this indicates that Satan affects the person (*ibid*: 16).

Samaaha discusses some of his cases. He divides them according to the "degree of harm caused by Satan." He mentions four kinds of satanic afflictions, which differ in the degree of consciousness and control sick persons have over their bodies and actions. Health then is a matter of having control. Sickness is a process of losing that control when an external agent takes over and directs the actions of the sick person (*ibid*: 16–17). My interpretation is that control may have infiltrated this discourse from a Freudian origin but it could also be an originally traditional idea that is further emphasized in present-day society.

Samaaha announces that the philosophy of his treatment aims at "liberating human behavior from the control of Satan, to the degree where individuals act according to their own will and reason and thus become obedient as required" (*ibid*: 23). Who exactly Satan is becomes clear through the second aim of therapy. It is a force that operates against the will of the person concerned (*ibid*: 23). Recovery is realized when satanic behavior is "reduced to its weakest point or made to disappear completely" (*ibid*: 23). Furthermore, the aim of Quranic therapy is "the development of human behavior through training and cultivation to realize compliance to all legitimate commands" (*'awāmir sha'iyyah*) (*ibid*). The Arabic word *sharᶜiyya* has a double meaning. As Talal Asad (1993) notes, "while it connotes the general modern sense of "legitimate," it derives from the specific Islamic concept of "the divinely sanctioned law-and-morality" (*al-shariᶜa*) (*ibid*: 212). Samaaha keeps this term undefined, which leads to ambiguity. He stresses that recovery is realized when "the individual grows up to the way of obedience until he becomes totally immune and preserved" (Samaaha 1996: 23).

Are these definitions part of a spiritual healing traditionally known in Egyptian society? Is the sheikh performing religious therapy? Alternatively, is he reflecting the dominant discourse that requires individuals to exercise conscious control over their bodies? Does his treatment include surviving elements from Stoic moral philosophy with its emphasis on self-mastery? Clearly, elements from various traditions are present in Samaaha's language and thought. These elements have been pieced together to fit the present purpose of maintaining and restoring health in both the individual and collective sense.

Samaaha calls himself a Quranic therapist (*mu'ālig bi al-qur'ān*). In some of the newspaper clippings he is called Sheikh Samaaha. The traditional anthropological subject of a spiritual healer whose power consists in the aura around his charismatic figure is different from Samaaha. Traditionally, anthropologists have described healers who used to derive authority from their texts and other means that they tend to keep secret (see for example Frankenberg 1976). One newspaper article (*Al-Ahram* 12.9.1990) talks about him as a thirty-eight-year-old accountant. The article implies that his power of healing comes solely from the Quran, rather than from Samaaha himself. Samaaha says that he is no more than a means of healing. The power of the Quran is mediated too by al-Azhar. Samaaha includes a permit from al-Azhar to publish this guide for therapists.

Furthermore, Samaaha has not inherited the gift of healing from his family. He also did not learn it from an apprenticeship. He developed his knowledge and reputation throughout his study at al-Azhar, and during his healing activities. He describes some of those activities carried out in his home and other cases to support the idea that the Quran has healing power. The healer himself declares that laypersons can perform Quranic therapy. They and their patients only have to *believe* in the Quran for the therapy to be effective. The pamphlet is addressed to those people who are interested in learning or developing their healing capacities by reading the Quran and other scholarly works listed in Samaaha's guide.

Samaaha's text is a modern manual. However, it serves to reinforce the authority of an originally powerful text, the Quran. This is a process where one form of spiritual healing is reorganized and transformed. It aims at creating and maintaining independent subjects whose health has been related to the notion of control. The belief that the Quran has the power of healing is maintained under the auspices of an allegedly legitimate state and propagated along with modern biomedicine.

Samaaha also engages with psychiatrists. He attaches his debates with them in the newspaper clippings section. Psychiatrists who debate with the sheikh do not entirely agree with his methods. One psychiatrist addresses the sheikh: "your method is one therapeutic method accepted [in psychiatry] to treat hysterical functional diseases which have no physical basis. As such, it is exactly like our method even though the style in each case is different. Each one of us is moving in a different way: you are using a religious method, and we are using a scientific way, but both of us rely on notions of revelation" (cited in Samaaha: 164).

PSYCHIATRY: A CONTINUATION OF SPIRITUAL HEALING?

Many authors call spiritual illnesses or heart illnesses "illnesses of the soul" (*al-'amrāḍ al-nafsiyya*) (e.g., Abdallah 1993; Samaaha 1996). Simultaneously, the word "*nafsiyya*" (adjective from *nafs*, soul) is also the translation for the word psychological. Psychology is translated in modern Arabic as *'ilm al-nafs* (literally, science of the soul) where *al-nafs* is conceptualized in connection with modern definitions of health and illness. There is a relationship between the two coexisting meanings of *al-nafs*: *al-nafs* as a concept with roots in local culture, and *al-nafs* as a concept used in a modern discipline. Gamal Abul'azaayem, a physician and psychiatrist, discusses these ideas in a pamphlet entitled *The Quran and Psychological Health* (*al-qur'ān wa al-ṣiḥḥah al-nafsiyyah*, 1994). This pamphlet is an interesting example of cultural translation where modern disciplinary knowledge is introduced into local culture and then used by biophysical power. The author uses psychological concepts, originally devised to produce docile bodies, characteristic of modern society. Next, he connects these concepts with local traditional notions. The result is a composite form of knowledge that does not duplicate its constituents.

On the back cover, Abul'azaayem notes that in his years at Cairo University medical school, he has been "particularly concerned with connections between the Quran and medical and psychological sciences." This interest has been "assisted by his family background which helped him to memorize the Quran and to read its different interpretations with the guidance of a relative who is an Imam and scholar." Being "a member and colleague of the Royal College of Psychological Medicine in London" indicates his connection to western medicine.[2] He describes his life as "rich in social, medical and religious activities." He lists organizations, journals, and conferences in which he has either participated or initiated. Such descriptions are powerful in local terms. The back cover also includes the author's picture. He wears a white shirt and looks to be around sixty years old. He has a dark spot on his forehead, a sign of piety. Such a spot develops because of repeated prayers. Abul'azaayem's self-introduction represents the way in which many modernist intellectuals seek to establish their power in society. They emphasize their modern knowledge, but more importantly, they demonstrate that this knowledge has its roots in Muslim culture.

Abul'azaayem's pamphlet consists of reflections on Quranic verses that he interprets in connection to individual and social health. The assumption is that "many facts of human psychology published in the West have roots in the Quran" (*ibid*: 3). The author argues that the nervous system is mentioned in the Quran by allusion. He explains the relationship between the nervous system and the notion of *al-nafs*. He stresses the relevance of the "Quran to human psychological life in all stages of development" (*ibid*). He further describes a "relationship between various religious duties in Islam and an individual's psychological health in fields of prevention and therapy" (*ibid*). Finally, he extends these reflections onto society and explains their implications for the social and political organization of health services from an Islamic perspective.

Underlying Abul'azaayem's ideas is an assumption that religion and science have a similar approach to life and health. As such, science should be employed to unravel an eternal truth that the multitudes of Quranic meanings are believed to have. These meanings need to be constantly reinterpreted in order to arrive at useful ideas. However, what practical ideas does the author have in mind, and how do these ideas represent the political agenda underlying this connection between science and the Quran? At the beginning of the pamphlet the author quotes the following verse,

> And every human being's destiny We have tied to his neck; and on the Day of Resurrection We shall bring forth for him a record which he will find wide open; [and he will be told:] Read this thy record! Sufficient is thine own self today to make out thine account (*sura al-'isra'*: 13).

In the Quran a "Human being's destiny" is described by the word *ta'ir*, which means bird, or flying creature. The Quranic use of this term refers to a pre-Islamic practice where people used to foretell the future or their fortune from the direction in which birds flew (Asad 1980). The reference here is to human beings' choices, which they consciously make throughout their lives. Abul'azaayem argues that *ta'ir* indirectly refers to the nervous system during the embryonic stages of an individual's life where the nervous system looks like a structure with two wings (*ibid*: 8). What is the connection between the nervous system and the cultural concept of *al-nafs*? The author asserts that *al-nafs* is what occurs in the brain and the whole nervous system. It is the force that orchestrates billions of living cells. Science, he proceeds, has detected waves of energy circulating in all cells. After several pages in which he quotes the Quran and provides drawings of the nervous system to further substantiate his interpretations, he concludes, these currents are "the personality of the human being, or his characteristic energies or the mode of his responses, or what the product of what we call the human soul (*nafs al-'insān*)" (*ibid*: 14).

Based on another Quranic verse, Abul'azaayem argues that this energy acts like a watchman (*raqib*) on the acts, thoughts, and feelings of individuals throughout their life. In a manner that echoes philosophical descriptions of pervasive technologies of surveillance in modern society, the watchman as mentioned in the Quran is "closer to individuals than their neck vein" (*ibid*: 18), and will report those actions to God on the day of Resurrection. The records will not disappear upon death. God will retrieve them. To show that recovering past actions is possible, the author mentions an example of similar operations conducted by scientists. He notes that techniques have been developed to restore lost memories (*ibid*: 20).

According to Abul'azaayem and others who quote the Quran (e.g., Samaaha 1996) *al-nafs* is a force, a potential originally shaped by God. It is given content during individuals' lives. In each individual *al-nafs* is composed of two conflicting forces: (1) *nafs* forces individuals to commit sin; (2) *nafs* forces them to be virtuous. The following verse is quoted by Abul'azaayem to indicate a conflict that exists inside each individual.

> Consider the human self, and how it is formed in accordance with what it is meant to be; and how it is imbued with moral failings as well as with consciousness of God! To a happy state shall indeed attain he who causes this [self] to grow in purity; and truly lost is he who buries it [in darkness] (*sura al-Shams*, 7–10).

This understanding of *al-nafs* in the Quran includes the physical body as interpreted by Muhammad Asad (1980) who recognizes other meanings of this term. However, generally the term refers to "the human self or personality as a whole: that is, being composed of a physical body and that inexplicable life-essence loosely described as the "soul" (*ibid*: 954). Abul'azaayem's interpretation reflects this understanding when he states that spiritual practices shape the body. He maintains that Islamic duties engender obedience and good conduct and thus help the virtuous force to override the sinful one. Proper Islamic education, Abul'azaayem argues, establishes an Islamic community where values of obedience (*al-ṭā'ah*), discipline (*al-ta'addub*), patience (*al-ṣabr*) and forbearance (*al-ḥilm*) are prevalent. These practices lead to regulation of desires (*ḍabṭ al-shahawāt*). The final aim of this system, as seen by Abul'azaayem, is to create an homogeneous, smoothly and effectively functioning society. The family is supposed to continue the education pursued by society. It needs to reinforce values that "aim at taming the soul and leading it to maturity" (*ibid*: 50). All these factors are essential for quieting (*taskīn*) destructive motives such as the sexual ones. For Abul'azaayem, all these objectives are embodied in the five pillars of Islam. He explains how these pillars inscribe the above values into the individual soul. This process, he assumes, will eventually translate onto the structure of the group (*ibid*: 14).

Abul'azaayem's ideas echo Samaaha's main premises. Particularly, he argues that *'imān*, which is another term for the concept of *yaqīn* used by Samaaha, has immense utility in healing. Thus, each "culture should benefit from its spiritual potentials by all means available" (*ibid*: 83). For him the concept of *'imān* needs to operate through the mosque which is the "place of worship . . . center for education . . . and health care" (*ibid*: 84). The mosque provides psychiatric therapy, as he himself does in a mosque/clinic complex. The mosque where he practices is named after his relative, Imam Mohammed Maadi Abul'azaayem. This mosque is part of a larger complex including a health dispensary, youth center, library, family-support center, kindergarten, nursery school, drug rehabilitation unit, and classrooms for after-school lessons.

This mosque is not unique. Many similar complexes are maintained by Islamic philanthropic organizations and provide social and health services for lower-income groups. Morsy (1988) describes these institutions as part of the global socioeconomic system. She maintains that they are employed to promote a global biomedical hegemonic culture. However, this does not preclude that these institutions also have intellectual, social, and economic programs, which are relatively autonomous. It is misleading to assume that these programs are totally driven by outside forces and thus only realize the objectives of a global economy. This assumption is based on an understanding that the power of that system is unalterable. It implies that the results of interactions between forces of the global market, which are themselves operating within heterogeneous contexts, are predetermined.

Furthermore, it is important to identify the social groups involved in these services, and their political ends. These complex questions need to be researched separately. I argue that these groups appropriate different medical resources and reinvent them. This reinvention involves translating various medical statements into culturally relevant meanings. These meanings are put into action by local institutions. The processes of translation and implementation need to demonstrate how different medical ideas are relevant to contemporary health and social problems. There is no indication that the processes of reworking different medical ideas will ever produce one or more homogeneous framework for practice. That individuals involved in these processes continuously seek to realize uniformity should indicate that uniformity has not yet been achieved.

Abul'azaayem talks about his clinic/mosque as a social-religious-psychological center (*al-markiz al-'igtimā'i al-dīni al-nafsi*). A research project conducted by this center illustrates the way processes of fusing different elements into a workable unit occur. Abul'azaayem mentions this research project in order to illustrate that therapies provided at his center are highly efficacious, especially when compared to those provided by "ordinary clinics" (*'iyādāt 'ādiyya*). Ordinary clinics, according to Abul'azaayem, use only chemical drugs and standardized psychiatric methods. The research involved applying therapies on 120 individuals addicted to opium. The individuals were divided into two groups. One group underwent treatment at an "ordinary clinic" and the other at Abul'azaayem's clinic. He stresses that his therapy is far more successful than that of the other clinics. Abul'azaayem's explanation of the results of the study and the difference between the two places is very interesting. He thinks his group was more successfully treated because faith (*'imān*) was part of the therapy. *'Imān* was also present in the therapeutic team of psychiatrist, social worker, and preacher. Abul'azaayem adds that the practitioners were chosen because of their piety (*ibid*: 86).

Therapy was administered immediately after group prayers at the mosque. The center showed addicts videotapes that "illustrate God's eminence in order to further their faith" (*ibid*: 87). The reliance on the notion of *'imān* links Abul'azaayem to Samaaha. The difference between them lies in the method and type of combination between chemical drugs and the Quran. Their basic premises are related. Another difference lies in the fact that Abul'azaayem extends his ideas to include society as a whole. Referring to mosque-based therapy, Abul'azaayem continues, "the same should be done in the family, the school, the social club, and all other places and gatherings" (*ibid*: 87). Thus, individual and social health can be realized. However, how can individual and social well-being be maintained? Individual health is represented by the soul, which is the product of the energy flowing in the nervous system. The society's health is represented by state of balance that can be achieved if there is a good leadership. He argues that the leadership of society is its central nervous system: "if those in government live up to their responsibilities, they would succeed" (*ibid*: 114). Then Abul'azaayem identifies illnesses that might afflict the body of society:

> Society is the product of its individuals' energies. It displays its individuals' various features and attributes. It is healthy when they are healthy. Otherwise, society will be disorderly. Leaders are the central nervous system of society, if they live up to their responsibilities, they will succeed. If they are easily provoked, hasty, and afflicted by doubt and fear, then all these qualities will reflect on the behavior of the whole group, which will suffer and then try to change its conditions. If it fails it will surrender and become weaker and be dominated by the spirit of weakness and defeat" (*ibid*: 114).

This is a political statement based on biophysical-religious grounds. It illustrates the end result of a description that started with the microcosm of the nervous cell and ended with the macrocosm of the social being. Does Abul'azaayem imply that since society also has a nervous system (its leadership), it must also have a *nafs*, and this *nafs* is accountable before God? Abul'azaayem does not pursue these ideas. Nevertheless, his ideas lead to such a result and imply a critique inspired by physiology, psychology, and religion. Subsequently, it is not surprising that at the end of his pamphlet he calls for political actions based on these ideas. He calls for a democratic society whose government is inspired by the Islamic political concept of *shūrā* (consultation) between the ruler and the ruled. He believes that this combination can eventually produce a society healthier than the existing one (*ibid*: 114).

Abul'azaayem's ideas illustrate how concepts with roots in tradition, such as the ones used by Samaaha and Abdallah, continue to be used by practitioners of modern science. In this process, concepts are not radically changed.

They are reorganized. Their connection to older styles of reasoning remains open. Therefore, their use continues to evoke diverse meanings in different contexts. Moreover, Abul'azaayem is undertaking an endeavor where concepts with roots and power in popular knowledge are relocated and used to disseminate modern disciplinary knowledge. More importantly, they are used to realize a new kind of interactive governance. These concepts are recreated as they are employed by a far more pervasive discourse promoted by the state, science, and religion. In the present case, the concept of *al-nafs* has been vitalized in a completely new way by including it into the discourse on biophysical power. The influence of powerful hegemonic discourses is evident in uses of *al-nafs* to explain illnesses in Cairo. Innumerable pathological states of being are explained as resulting from a *ḥāla nafsiyya* (a condition of the soul). Statements such as spiritual condition (*ḥāla ruuhiyya*) or mental condition (*ḥāla 'aqliyya*) however are never used in everyday life to explain pathological conditions. I argue that the concepts of *al-rūḥ* and *al-'aql* have been marginalized in the process of promoting and disseminating the notion of *al-nafs* through modern science.

Finally, Abul'azaayem's way of conceptualizing health and illness might appear contradictory and improvised. His contradictions and ceaseless search for solutions for everyday problems underlie the development of his ideas as a practitioner. They also reflect his interest in power. His ideas have roots in modern education, society, and historical culture. These elements motivate him to criticize both modern life and society represented by its institutions: "we should sow the seeds of *al-'imān* in this desert called modern life. The same applies to the family, school, social club, and all places of gathering" (*ibid*: 87).

CONCLUSION

The above pamphlets present ideas and practices illustrating and confirming the arguments presented in the introduction to this study, including the plurality of the Egyptian medical system that seeks to maintain a holistic meaning of *ṣiḥḥah* or correctness. They lend support to the idea that the Egyptian tradition shows a strong sense of continuity by viewing the body as intricately connected to the mind, spirit, and soul as traditionally defined. However, questions that remain to be addressed include, first, whether such understandings relate to everyday practice. In other words, how are they manifest in people's search for help and, more critically, in the processes of evaluating available therapies and the relevance of these to existing physical and moral problems? These questions are dealt with in the next two chapters on the family and the social syndrome of '*iḍḍaghṭ*.

NOTES

1. See *al-munjid fi all-lugha wa al-a'alaam*.

2. Whether this is true or not is not of particular relevance here. What matters is the fact that the author feels it is important to show a connection to a western country when he introduces himself.

2

Family Life, Health, and Illness

Examples from *Būlāq Abul'ela*

It is early morning in *Būlāq Abul'ela*, a residential, commercial and industrial quarter of Cairo. The noise of many metal workshops has already started, vegetable stalls, grocery stores, coffee shops, food vendors, bakers and barbers' shops are opening. Around small stalls and vendors, queues of children and grown-ups wait to buy fresh *fūl*, an extremely popular morning dish of spiced fava beans. In some of the small restaurants, men are eating *fūl* with pickles and drinking dark sweet tea. Others sit and chat in cafés. They will stay longer if they are unemployed and starting another slow day; some hope to be picked for a short spell of employment. On the corners, women place crates of vegetables and fruits out for sale. Itinerant vendors sell plastic dishes, aluminum pots, plastic slippers, and chicks. In the unpaved alleys groups of boys and girls walk to school carrying their colorful bags. Well-dressed men and women hurry to their office jobs. Everybody has to maneuver between cars and small trucks. A brand new Mercedes passes a thirty-year old Fiat. Horse-drawn carriages intermingle with the traffic.

This scene is a common one in many residential areas, especially those Cairenes call "*al-'ahyaa' al-sha'biyyah*" (popular quarters) where the majority of the city's population lives. Although *al-sha'biyya* literally means that the quarter is inhabited by "people," when Cairenes use this expression they have in mind at least two meanings: first, the place is inhabited by groups with incomes lower than those of quarters such as Zamalek, whose villas and high rise buildings stand across the Nile to the west of *Būlāq*, and second it is *taqlidi* or *baladi* (traditional, or indigenous). A closer look at *Būlāq*, however, reveals complexities that the apparently economic class based term of *sha'biyya* excludes and the term *baladi* does not represent. The term *sha'biyya* does not further specify the sociological or economic characteristics of the people in the above scene, which implies that several economic classes live in *Būlāq*. Likewise, the term *baladi* is used by different people with different purposes and interests. The lower classes, for example, use it to affirm their belonging to the nation. For them it implies the culturally formative nature of their practices. The upper classes use it as a symbol for what they perceive to be the cultural core of the nation. On other occasions, however, the latter classes use the term to point to practices they consider "backward," "old-fashioned," or "inefficient" and which do not fit into the modern way of life.

Early (1993), who studied *Būlāq* in the 1970s, uses the term *baladi* to mean a "total way of life-style" (*ibid*: 67). For her this means patterns of acting, speaking, and conducting different affairs of life that are distinguishable from what she calls *afrangi*, which refers to lifestyles that are seen as foreign, western, and modern, depending on the context, or belonging to the upper class. Elsewhere, however, she argues that this opposition is not totally exclusive. Some wealthy merchants choose to continue living in *baladi* quarters next to their warehouses, while low-income individuals try to imitate life styles and consumption patterns of upper-income westernized groups (*ibid*: 51). I hold that this is enough to indicate that the dichotomy of *baladi* and *afrangi* involves processes of negotiation and change that suggest more complex lifestyles or ways of acting. In the study of health and illness that follows, I assume that various ways of maintaining health are parts of a larger field of discursive practice that is continuously changing. Within this field, specific elements from different origins are involved in processes of interaction that occur under a variety of ever-evolving social and economic circumstances. In this interactive structure the very dichotomy of *baladi* and *afrangi*, including their anthropological descriptions, is a discursive practice connected to power relations: as such, it is not simply a tool but a subject for analysis.

Health practices in Egypt have long been a subject for historical and anthropological studies. They have been viewed as pluralistic systems of medical thought (Gran 1979), or as parts of dominant religious or philosophical ideologies (Bürgel 1976). Other studies analyze health practices as products of interaction or historical "clashes" between different theories of disease (Kuhnke 1990: 1–6, 153–166). Studies focusing on the different ways abstract theories are circulated and used by different groups have only just begun to emerge. Inhorn's (1994) study of infertility and gender in Alexandria analyzes medical practices rooted in ancient Egypt, Unani-Greek-Islamic medicines, and modern biomedicine. Inhorn argues that to understand current concepts of procreation,

> it is necessary to understand the historically situated, cultural construction of reproductive knowledge in Egypt and the ways in which such knowledge has been transmuted and translated into quotidian discourse over time (*ibid*: 53).

Similarly, I am concerned with the use of multiple health care resources in contemporary Cairo. My goal is to situate the contemporary health practices of individuals in the historical and contemporary social, economic, and cultural landscape of *Būlāq*, which is one of the city's central quarters. Diverse health resources in *Būlāq* exist in conditions characterized by a perceived decline in public services, a worsening of living conditions, and a continuous decrease in the opportunities for individuals to find employment and live independently. This situation has given the family an overriding importance. I aim at exploring the impact of these conditions on the meanings of health, illness, the individual, and the social body.

As for health perceptions, I argue that the health of the individual body is a function of the working of the social relations surrounding it. In this context, all individuals have their families as their best "therapeutic management group." They routinely exchange medical information with other members as well as with friends, neighbors, and other people accessed through family networks. Information exchanged involves therapies that combine elements from biomedicine, humoral theory, and spiritual healing where all are perceived as interrelated, although they might operate differently. Other cases illustrate the point that health and illness are essentially parts of one *single field*; that is, a vision of life that cannot simply be divided into different aspects such as the physical, the social, the psychological, or the emotional. *Health is regarded not as a mere medical category but as a parameter reflecting the material and social prosperity of the social unit in which individuals live. In short, health ultimately means life*. In conclusion, I would agree with the widely circulated argument that people should not be regarded as agents separated from their families as they may be conceptualized in standard biomedical practice. Kleinman et al. (1994) would argue that the latter would exclude complex "processes that inscribe history and social relations onto the body." In addition, I would argue that such separation reduces the individuals' socialized consciousness about health and pain to mere biological categories. Furthermore, in the case of *Būlāq* in particular and Cairo in general individuals express their whole life, including their conditions, in medical terms.All sorts of systems, the Greek-Islamic or modern biomedicine, are no less than forms of living, and some individuals require treatment of some kind. However, some others simply do not. These conditions presuppose relations with family, friends, neighbors, and co-workers. They are constantly linked with ideas and feelings about society as a whole; these feelings are present as essential constituents. In essence, life as such certainly presupposes something that is much wider than the individual body.

Furthermore, I argue that therapies resulting from complex social, moral, emotional, and practical evaluations and combining elements from different health resources produce "amalgams" of therapeutic methods that identify with the experience of the individuals involved, and not necessarily with any of the "systems" of knowledge employed in the therapeutic process. These "composite" therapies sought and applied by people are ever-shifting structures of knowledge based on practical, aesthetic, and moral considerations. These considerations can never be described by the sociological concept of "negotiation," which is also used by anthropologists who celebrate various forms of transactionalist theories. These considerations are guided by issues that are not commoditized or objectified and thus are very difficult to treat as parts of a business deal. I would therefore suggest viewing them as complex processes of moral valuation.

The structure of medical care services is obviously dominated by biomedicine, which nevertheless has acquired powerful political and religious idioms. Powerful institutions such as the state and the mosque provide these services. This domination, however, does not necessarily entail all the therapeutic activities being eventually determined by biomedical explanatory models. There are at least two reasons limiting this determination. First, biomedicine is not equally distributed among all the social groups. Second, even among those who have full access to biomedical facilities, the physical treatment they obtain provides a specific kind of solution to their problems. People always view these problems as manifestations of larger and more complex adverse conditions affecting their social and emotional lives that require them to incorporate biomedicine with other healing methods. In doing so, and given their low incomes, people rely on reasoning that is only partially shaped by the concepts underlying the above resources, including Islamic literary sources and the media connected to them. People rely primarily on what can best be called *practical reason.* This reason is dynamic: it is shaped by the immediate concerns of the body and more diffused cultural concerns. As such, people weigh up the therapies provided at different health facilities in a complex manner: their *general well-being* as individuals as well as families is always being considered. Here is the connection with the home-based therapeutic activities. Biomedical therapies are combined with herb-based therapies as well as religious or spiritual remedies. None of these therapies can be seen as separate or exclusive. Health behavior in *Būlāq* best matches Worsley's (1982) insight into medicine as a resource rather than a system. His description of health seekers as "pragmatic, flexible and experimental" applies to the vast majority, if not all, of the individuals in *Būlāq*. The aim of patients, as Worsley also argues, is not to evaluate certain therapies or theories but rather to recover from pain and distress and by any means.

This chapter consists of two parts. In the first part I describe the landscape of *Būlāq* and how it is composed of continuing elements from different historical periods. Then I describe various living conditions, including population size and density and the quality of housing. Then I include an overview of the health resources in *Būlāq*. In the second part I explore various life conditions of my study group, which is made up of ten families. After a note on the way I approached the families and established a rapport with them, I focus on the families' living spaces, social ties, age structures, education, and employment. Then I discuss three situations that involve management of health and illness within the structure of the family. Finally, I discuss the views expressed in these situations, which although unrepresentative, illustrate widely shared principles of health care specific to the social setting of *Būlāq*. The case studies illustrate people's perceptions of their health status and their major concern with matters related to keeping good health.

THE PAST IN THE PRESENT

In the current administrative division, *Būlāq* is part of west Cairo and forms a triangular shaped area bounded on the northeast by al-Sabtiya Street, which separates it from another low-income residential quarter called Gazirat Badran and the populous quarter of Shubra. In a westerly direction *Būlāq* ends in a group of glittering modern high-rise buildings that separate its dark yellow sun-dried brick buildings from the eastern bank of the Nile. These tall buildings include the Nile Hilton, the National Bank of Egypt, the World Trade Center–Cairo, the Foreign Ministry, and the building of the National Radio and Television. They stand between *Būlāq* and Corniche el-Nil, formerly a favorite spot for afternoon walks for people from *Būlāq* and other areas. The east of the southern side of *Būlāq* is bounded by the busy street of al-Galaa' which houses the headquarters of *Al-Ahram* and *Akhbar al-Youm*, the two major national newspapers. Further west of Al-Galaa' street is the formerly colonial "westernized" quarter of Garden City that developed during the nineteenth century along the Nile, and was initially a neighborhood for the foreign administration and later for the rising Egyptian elite. To the southeast of Garden City lies "Eastern" Old Cairo for which *Būlāq* used to be the link to the Nile.

Abu-Lughod's (1971) city map that depicts Eastern Cairo in opposition to westernized sections of the city should be reconsidered in light of the growing similarities between Cairo's older divisions. In the fifty years following the end of the colonial state, Cairo has grown into one "cultural unit" (*ibid*: 208–209). This unity was promoted by a nationalist discourse aimed at creating a homogenized capital that could stand for a unified nation despite evident class and ethnic differences. Divisions between the "poor" and the "rich," the "indigenous" and the "western," the "traditional" or "*baladi*" and the "modern" have been pushed to the back of the populist rhetoric of post-colonial governments for the benefit of a discourse that presented all these categories as parts of one metropolis, lately announced as Greater Cairo (*al-Qahira al-Cobra*). This metropolis is seen to combine tradition and modernity, a civilization that is able to "Egyptianize" foreign elements. The term *sha'biyya* (popular),[1] which includes different classes under one category, is no less than a manifestation of the same discourse.

Contemporary *Būlāq* is distinguishable from both the older and the newer parts of Cairo. It is located outside the walls of Islamic Cairo. Its geographical history starts in the mid-thirteenth century when the Nile retreated and revealed an inhabitable area (Hanna 1983). At first, during the Mamluk period, wealthy notables inhabited the emerging land. In the middle of the fifteenth century a port was established on the newly formed riverbank of *Būlāq*. The port remained in use during successive periods, including the Ottoman occupation, and it was in use when Napoleon's army invaded Cairo in the late eighteenth century. Shortly afterwards, when Mohammed Ali Pasha, the powerful and ambitious Sultan of Egypt, came to power in 1805, *Būlāq* witnessed a period of great transformation during his forty-year reign. The Pasha's modernizing economic and military projects, the largest in the whole region at the time, had a far-reaching impact on Egypt and other areas in the Sudan, Syria, and the Arabian Peninsula. Along with massive military development, the Pasha launched major agricultural and economic reforms and industrial projects. During that time, *Būlāq*'s port served as the main connection between the Pasha's government and the outside world. Subsequently, tens of factories and commercial firms were established around the port. The factories included two lathe workshops, eighty iron workshops, a wool factory, textile and spinning factories, and the first printing press (Early 1993: 30–31). Although abandoned, the printing press building still stands, next to the overpowering tower of the World Trade Center. Remnants of some of the commercial firms are still visible, several being used as warehouses. They are called *Wikaalaat* (pl. of *Wikaalah* or commercial agency), establishments with architectural characteristics typical of *Būlāq* (Hanna 1983).

Būlāq was among the first quarters in Cairo to have modern medical facilities including one clinic, because it was one of the most densely populated areas in the city (Kuhnke 1990). Kuhnke mentions that those facilities were concerned with overseeing the public health. They provided smallpox vaccination for children and took the steps necessary to prevent outbreaks. The clinic was staffed by physicians who were supposed to provide free treatment especially to the poor (*ibid*: 142). It is partly for this reason that people in *Būlāq* show considerable familiarity with modern medicine: it has been available in the area for some time.

It is true that many of the residents are not aware of this history. Nevertheless, it is also true that all *Būlāq*is continue to live in spaces shaped by history, which is incarnated in structures such as mosques, the most prominent and continuing feature of *Būlāq*. Many of the mosques in *Būlāq* encompass shrines where *ṣūfi* leaders are buried. I argue that such spaces point to local histories that are remembered and transmitted by most of the residents. There is at least one mosque and a shrine in every main alley. The second part of *Būlāq*'s name, *Abul'ela*, refers to a *ṣūfi* figure who lived and observed his prayers in a local mosque that is still functioning and carries his name. The mosque continues to receive great respect and material support in the form of donations from both the government and the general public. This and other shrines are visited by men and women who seek the help of the living spirit of the *wali* (saint).

Shrines and mosques are not the only features distinguishing *Būlāq* from more recent neighborhoods that have mushroomed around Cairo due to an increased influx from the countryside following the 1952 revolution. It is true that residents of the recent neighborhoods also come from rural backgrounds similar to those of people of *Būlāq*. However, *Būlāq*'s connection to historic Cairo remains much stronger due to the fact that it has been included in the older city for several centuries. This is evident in the physical layout of *Būlāq*: old herb shops and old public baths can be found alongside biochemical pharmacies; spiritual healing is available alongside modern biomedical facilities such as clinics, which are sometimes attached to and sponsored by mosques. The question here is not to identify the origins of these juxtaposed elements, but to demonstrate how they all constitute a continuing and interacting past that forms present *Būlāq*.

Industrial activity in *Būlāq* continued throughout the twentieth century. An observer during the 1930s recorded that on his way through the area "hundreds of small dark workshops echo with the noise of hammers on red hot iron and on copper pans" (Leprette 1939: 253). However, in the last few decades large-scale national industrial projects have dominated the market, and traditional businesses are no longer the mainstay they once were. The result is that *Būlāq* has become a slum for people who had to stay there because they could not afford to move, rather than being populated by people who stayed for reasons related to the availability of jobs.

In the 1970s Early (1993) noticed that there were still wealthy merchants living what she calls a "*baladi* life-style in elegant, crumbling apartments deep in the back lanes" (*ibid*: 33). Given how difficult it has become to find new living space in Cairo, some of those people still lived in *Būlāq* in the 1990s. Expensive cars, big funeral processions, and lavish wedding parties indicate that the class is still represented in the neighborhood. Among the poorer classes it is rumoured that it is this class of people who have so far prevented the government from giving way to various landlords interested in clearing the older buildings to make way for profitable projects such as upmarket tenement buildings, hotels, and shopping malls.

Superficially, the present *Būlāq* might look as though it has been totally merged into the city. Beneath the surface, however, class boundaries continue to be reproduced in a variety of almost invisible ways. Early (1993) is right in arguing that

> Since the wealthy . . . have lost the privilege of geographic isolation, they distance themselves in other ways. Cognitive boundaries have become rigid as territorial lines have relaxed in response to the population crunch and Nasserist policies of nationalisation and public sector development (*ibid*: 40).

The same cognitive maps operate between residents of the old tenements of *Būlāq* and the massive tower of the World Trade Centre–Cairo, located a few footsteps from their impoverished dwellings. Children from *Būlāq* have to disguise themselves when they go for a tour of the tower, where they gaze at shiny stores filled with goods with unimaginable price tags. They choose their best clothes in order to fool the security guards at the main doors. *Būlāq*is are aware of such divisions despite the visible evidence that their neighborhood has physically merged into the metropolis.

*Būlāq*is are aware that their neighborhood has many problems associated with the lack of proper government services. Many of them demand the sanitation system be upgraded and extended to the whole quarter. They also demand that drinking water should reach higher buildings where people on the upper floors have to wait hours to fill a bucket. *Būlāq*is are also aware that these problems are the signs of a low-income group. Curiously, however, many of them refuse to call them signs of "poverty." A combined sense of honor and hope prevents people from labelling themselves as "poor" since poverty is associated with defeat (*ghulb*, adj. *ghalbaan*). Honor is the reason people work or look for jobs that enable them to support themselves. Hope is a constant force that motivates people to appropriate and adapt those indicators that appear on wealthier people seen on the street or the TV.

These problems related to success engender ill health for *Būlāq*is. As for overcrowding, the major influx of the population took place around the time of World War II: these newcomers were from the countryside. This influx continued throughout the following decades: Nasser's Cairo pulled many landless peasants to the city to look for jobs (Abu-Lughod 1971).[2] Waterbury (1978) quotes government sources that estimate the population density in *Būlāq* in 1966 to have been 74,716 persons per km^2. The total area of *Būlāq* is 2.7 km^2 (*ibid*: 180). This means that the population at that time was around

201,733 persons. This is almost midway between the most densely populated neighborhood of Bab el-Sha'raiyya, the highest rated at a density of 135,901 km^2, and the least densely populated area of Mataria at the fringes of Cairo which had 4,606 persons per km^2 (*ibid*: 180). Assuming that the growth rate of *Būlāq*'s population followed the rate of natural increase for the whole country, which is currently 1.98 percent (Population Reference Bureau 2000) and which has only decreased in the last few decades, we can roughly estimate that the population size of *Būlāq* increased between 1966 and 1996 to no less than 321,562 persons with a population density of 118,424 persons per km^2. This number might be higher because, as part of Cairo, *Būlāq* continued to receive new immigrants.

People of *Būlāq* live in buildings made of sun-dried brick that make up the sides of unpaved alleys (two to three meters wide) and lanes. What increases density is that the buildings, which often have adjacent walls, are two to six floors high. I carried out most of my participant observation research in *Būlāq el-Gidid* (or Modern *Būlāq*), a section located at the western edge of *Būlāq* that is composed of tenements of three to six floors. Dwellers of *Būlāq* el-Gidid live in apartments built in the 1920s and 1930s. These modern apartments are divided according to well-defined purposes. The size of the households in this section varies greatly, a factor that makes statistical figures too general to be useful. Furthermore, I noticed that the household size depends on the phase of the life cycle of the family. Economic constraints often prevent new generations from moving out. Some of the households consist of more than two generations and thus resemble extended families. Other households are composed of nuclear families, while some are made up of terminal families consisting of widows and children.

These three family structures differ from ideal anthropological types. In the case of the extended family, for example, the resources of the individual members are not totally shared. Each member keeps part of their income for future plans and projects such as marriage. On the other hand, individuals contribute to the living costs of the whole household. Other households that have nuclear families are not totally cut off from their parents' homes. The two nuclear families I include in this chapter are very well connected with their original family. They constantly exchange visits to celebrate religious holidays as well as events such as wedding parties, funerals, birthdays, and so forth.

Both sides feel obliged to provide help for each other, especially in times of crisis that sometimes require lending and borrowing money or hosting a relative for some time. Likewise, terminal families composed of widows and their children maintain their relations in material and emotional senses with the children who have moved out.

Social life in this section of the city requires people to creatively preserve their inherited values in contexts of diminished resources due to high rates of inflation, decreased job opportunities, and the withdrawal of state support. Simultaneously, the struggle for a hoped-for material reality linked with highly valued family life is complicated by values acquired from the mass media encouraging people to seek lucrative jobs at home and abroad. Most influential among all other messages spread by the media is the possibility of becoming rich very fast. Images and stories of the few who have made it and have moved to middle and upper income positions are disproportionately represented. Nevertheless, the standards of living that people aspire to have to confront the historical material realities into which they are born. An example is Ashraf who is in his mid-forties and has worked as a wage laborer for more than twenty-five years since completing his diploma. During this time he could not find a stable job that paid enough for him to marry, or "open a home" as many *Būlāq*is would describe the process of establishing a family. After he had traveled abroad and worked in several Arab countries his parents in *Būlāq* arranged for him to marry Samia. After marriage Samia lived with Ashraf's parents when he was away. Upon Ashraf's return for good he moved with Samia and their daughter to a small apartment on the roof of the building next to the one in which his parents live. The apartment was simply a large room that Ashraf managed to divide into different small rooms after obtaining permission from the owner. Ashraf's visitors see his name printed next to the bell on a well-painted door, which leads to the "living room" with a brand new TV set and tape recorder in its center. The living room is separated from Ashraf and Samia's bedroom, and from that of their daughter, by thin walls installed by Ashraf. Moreover, the amount of furniture squeezed into the tiny apartment includes a dining table and four chairs as well as a number of couches and two fans. On the walls there are posters that are copies of paintings. All these images reminded me of objects I saw in the homes of people belonging to higher income groups. Samia was proud of the fully automatic washing machine in the kitchen, an asset that every *sitti bait* (literally meaning house lady, which is the term for housewife) wishes to have. Ashraf's home is typical of many other houses that differ only in degree. His loyalty to his parents is represented by living next them to secure continuous visitation and incessant material and emotional support.

The private family life to which Ashraf aspires contrasts with another located just next door. Um Hamdi, sixty-five years old, and her daughter Hayam, twenty-eight years old, have been living in this section in their apartment, which is the top floor of an old sun-dried brick five-story building, for the last fifty years. Um Hamdi's apartment has two bedrooms, a separate kitchen, and a living room. It has been some time since the husband (Abu

Hamdi) died and the three sons (Hamdi, Khaled, and Ossaama) moved elsewhere in the city. The sons continue to support their mother and sister in various ways. As the size of the family became smaller, Um Hamdi and Hayam possessed more time and space for themselves. Therefore, they opened the living room to the outside to have access to the roof of the apartment below; in the hot summer afternoons Um Hamdi hangs out a plastic shade. Her many women friends in the neighborhood share the three old chairs and floor under the shade to exchange news or communicate other issues of interest. In addition, it is routine for Um Hamdi to call to the little boys playing down in the alley and ask them to buy her groceries in exchange for a little tip. It saves her going up and down the long and, at times, slippery staircases. The boys buy the groceries and place them in a basket hanging from a long string dangling from Um Hamdi's roof. Um Hamdi's balcony and basket are very common features of life in *Būlāq*. They represent a strong connection between the outside and inside spaces, and thus maintain ways of cooperation between neighbors (see al-Messiri 1977).

HEALTH RESOURCES

Just as *Būlāq* shows the influences of different periods of Egyptian history, it provides people with diverse ways of thinking and acting on their bodies in health and illness. In terms of health care facilities, *Būlāq* has two public hospitals, many private clinics, two mosque clinics, and many herb shops. Spiritual healing is also available through visits to the shrines found in many mosques. The utilization of these resources is, of course, conditioned by many factors such as affordability and perceived efficacy. Equally, if not more importantly, people have their own home-based therapeutic methods where they combine, compare, and evaluate different remedies from all the above resources.

The health facilities most accessible to people are those provided by the government hospitals which offer exclusively allopathic medical services. There are two major government hospitals in *Būlāq*. The first is a general hospital and the second is for obstetrics. The general hospital was built and maintained by the government shortly after the revolution in the 1950s. The shiny red color of its brick walls contrasts sharply with its poorly maintained interior and the old equipment. Every morning people, mostly women and children, form long queues before the hospital's gate. The hospital provides a wide range of curative services via junior and senior physicians who operate at the hospital on certain days of the week. The hospital has an inpatient clinic and several wards. The second hospital was built in the 1930s and its physical conditions are very similar to the general hospital. It has always been used by women from *Būlāq*, but also from other areas, which severely strains its services.

The second kind of medical facility is the mosque clinic, which also provides allopathic medicine. These are established, sponsored, and maintained by Islamic charitable societies. The condition of one of these clinics is similar to the government hospitals. It is housed on top of an old mosque and consists of two floors added at different stages. The clinic is managed by a local benevolent society supported by almsgiving at the mosque and donations from wealthy individuals who still live, or once lived, in *Būlāq*. The other clinic is in better condition. It is maintained by a much larger organization called "The Islamic-legal Society for the Co-operation of the Followers of the Quran and the Prophet's Traditions." Services at these clinics are similar to those provided by public hospitals except that they are nongovernment and attached to an Islamic discourse on medical care. I will discuss one such clinic, including the history and philosophy underlying its structure and services, in the next chapter. The clinic is presented as part of a continuing Islamic tradition represented by the Quran, the Prophet's traditions, and Islamic history. The principle that health care should be provided to the general public on an equitable basis is presented as originating in the moral mission of Islam. Furthermore, principles of modern science are reconstructed to demonstrate their roots in Islamic sacred texts such as the Quran, a reconstruction that supports the above moral and political mission.

The third medical facility in *Būlāq* is the *'iyādah* (plural *'iyādāt*, the Arabic term for a general practice) where allopathic medicine is also provided. Some of the *'iyādāt* in *Būlāq* are operated by several physicians with different specialties. An *'iyādah* is basically a private outpatient clinic that receives patients for physical examination and prescribes medicines dispensed at commercial pharmacies. All the *'iyādāt* in *Būlāq* are based in apartments with one or two nurses to help in routine work, such as the giving of injections. The nurse also helps with charging the patients for the physician's services. A typical *'iyādah* would have one room where visitors wait to see the doctor, and another for physical examinations, prescribing medicines, changing dressings, giving injections, etcetera. Some of the *'iyādāt* are kept neat and have new, and sometimes fancy, furniture. These are operated mostly by specialists who charge more than general practitioners. Most general practitioners' clinics are in poorer condition, having less space and furniture. The room for physical examinations usually has a couch and a desk in addition to few instruments used for basic physical examinations.

Herb shops and pharmacies are another source of health advice for many people in *Būlāq*. Herbs are widely perceived as being the original ancient source of those chemical medicines available at modern pharmacies. Knowledge of many herbs and chemical drugs is widely spread as a result of frequent visits to health specialists and readily available advice from friends and neighbors. Herb therapies are based on the humoral theory of disease, but it is important to grasp that people often combine herb-based therapies to biomedical ones as an examination of treatment reveals later in this chapter. Furthermore, many herbs in *Būlāq* are used to cure diseases that are originally defined by biomedical terms. Likewise, many biochemical pharmaceuticals are bought directly from pharmacies without prescription, and are used to treat complaints that include illnesses identified by humoral medicine. The line separating herb and biomedical therapies is always being crossed and recrossed, and cannot, in fact, be strictly defined—especially in the case of therapies conducted at home.

As for the cost of medical care, consultations at public hospitals are free but people have to pay for most of the medicines they are prescribed, although the cost is subsidized. Sometimes people are asked to buy the medicines at private pharmacies because the hospitals do not cover therapies for certain diseases. The cost of treatment at the mosque clinics is slightly higher. People have to pay three Egyptian pounds for the physical examination and sometimes have to buy the medicines prescribed independently at private pharmacies.[3] Payment for more special services is arranged separately. Slightly higher than the mosque clinic is the cost of visits to general practitioners who charge between five and ten Egyptian pounds per visit. Specialist physicians in private clinics, where people have to pay between twenty and fifty Egyptian pounds in order to see the doctor, charge the highest fees. The fees might increase, depending on the reputation of the physician and how specialized the examinations and therapies prescribed are. The price of therapies at herb shops varies enormously. Some herb-based therapies might be very expensive if they are rare, or are a mixture of many kinds of herbs.

At the public hospitals, people are aware of decreased state expenditure on medical care and as a result do not expect the therapies provided to be of much value. As for the mosque clinics, the religious principles underlying the work of these community-based institutions are not the only factors conditioning people's views about their services. It is true that religious views about health are widely circulated through various means such as the mosque preachers, TV, and the press, but people often see the mosque clinic as providing "second-rate" services undertaken by people who are not sufficiently qualified to deal with difficult problems. Many jokingly call the doctors working for the mosques as *kashkul*-doctors. *Kashkul* refers to the notepads that pupils use at school for miscellaneous notes. Likewise, *kashkul*-doctors claim the ability to cure a great variety of diseases, some of which are outside their field of expertise. A specialized *'iyādah* is the preferred kind of medical facility. All the people in my study group prefer to be examined and prescribed medicine by specialist physicians. Many are unhappy about the prices they pay for their visits, but they assume that a paid visit is always better than free government services, or those provided by mosque clinics at very low prices.

An important source for health-related information used at home are the media. TV sets and radios are situated at the center of most homes in *Būlāq*. Most cafés have TV sets turned on all the time. Medical knowledge, especially a biomedical perspective, is constantly presented in a variety of programs, often involving physicians. Newspapers also present a great variety of debates, advice, news, and commentaries on health issues, as I discuss in chapters 3 and 4. In addition to this information, people use the advice of their friends and relatives to come up with the best solutions within the limits of their financial resources, which they manage in an increasingly commercialized environment.

People are aware that high quality medical services are available in other parts of the city. They also know that these services are too expensive and provided for profit. In *Būlāq* the statement "medicine is a kind of business for profit" (*tigārah*) is routinely repeated by men and women from different age groups to point to the recent proliferation of facilities for private health care. A good example of this general feeling can be found in the words of Abla Afaaf, a woman in her late forties. Widowed and living with her two daughters, her husband passed away a few years ago after a long struggle with a stomach ulcer. In a cynical tone, she always made the pun: "Ahh, doctors! They are after five things that begin with the Arabic letter *ain*: *'iyādah* (clinic), *'arabiyya* (car), *'amārah* (building), *'izba* (rural estate) and *'arūsah* (bride).

Nevertheless medical care is mostly available in *Būlāq* through physicians who operate in their *'iyādāt* (private clinics) in the quarter and the mosque clinics. Certain physicians in *Būlāq* are preferred because "they treat people well." These "famous" physicians have been working in the area for many years. They have developed close relations with their patients; they know some of them personally. They are sometimes able to identify their families. Some of these practitioners were born and raised in *Būlāq*, and chose to have their clinics in the area where they already knew the inhabitants. Dr. Samir and his wife, Dr. 'Ula, who are both general practitioners are good examples of this kind of physician. Dr. Samir was born in *Būlāq el-Gidid* while his wife is from a different neighborhood. She moved to live and share his clinic after marriage. They both operate in one room and keep another room for patients to wait in; there a nurse tells the patients when to enter, does the office work, and charges patients as they walk out of the doctors' room. Despite this seemingly impersonal way, interacting as a member of the neighborhood, Dr. Samir speaks to many patients about their personal life, and exchanges news about their parents, brothers, and sisters. He accepts delayed payments from patients who cannot pay immediately after their visits. Physicians like Dr. Samir have helped indigenize biomedicine by linking it to local ways of interaction across professional lines. The mosque clinics also have gained respect for their services; many people have a great respect for them. The low quality of their clinical services is balanced out by the fact that they are introduced via a larger structure including an orphanage, a school, and free training programs that empower underprivileged groups. Biomedicine is inserted into a complex structure of inherited symbols. People respect the mosque clinic not through a purely clinical method of reasoning but a social and religious one.

Ultimately, the services provided are only medical and not concerned with other aspects affecting people lives. My argument is that inasmuch as medical resources shape people's experiences, they are also shaped through a process of negotiation and reworking that incorporates them into the larger worldview of the people who utilize them. This worldview guides people's performance when they try to meet their various physical, psychological, and social needs. In this context, the family plays a crucial role in maintaining the health of the individuals by linking the meanings of various illnesses and therapies to other events and sources of distress affecting their lives. It will shortly be clear that individuals are not separate agents, but subjects living out complex emotional and physical ties within their family structures.

FAMILIES IN *BŪLĀQ*

The main social unit in this neighbourhood is an individual household connected to a few others through close kinship relations or old relations of friendship. The former kind of relationship is much stronger than the latter. It is around parents, brothers, sisters, children, and grandchildren that the lives of people in *Būlāq* are organized. Individuals in this study are not viable as social or economic agents away from their roles as sons, daughters, fathers, mothers, and so on (see Hoodfar 1997; Watson 1992: 3–11). Family members keep close contact with each other when they have to share their space, food, money, and, in some cases, their clothes. Family relations lead them to share not only these objects, but other human "assets" including individuals' dreams and life projects such as marriage, study, and career ambitions. Fathers and mothers in this community often spend their lives trying to save for or set up a decent future for their children. Such a task takes enormous dedication. No wonder then that parents describe their children as parts of their bodies: mothers, for instance say their children are pieces from their hearts (*ḥitta min 'albi*) or, more intimately, their livers (*ḥitta min kibdi*).

Individuals and their sense of health and illness have thus a complex relation with various familial circumstances. In my meetings I aimed at focusing discussions on what I understood as "health-related questions." However, people always answered briefly about "physical health" *per se*. They quickly turned to other subjects such as a son failing in school, a daughter who had recently lost her job or another who has never found one, or a husband who is wasting money on a hopeless business. These preoccupations do not mean those individuals are not concerned with health questions, or that health does not occupy a central position in their lives. It means that the definition of health covers an area in which physical pain is connected to the themes they brought into the conversation. It means that proper functioning of the individual body is intrinsically connected to proper working of social relations.

The strongest commitment in the family is between parents and children. There is a time-honored custom in Egypt that requires parents to support children until they become old enough to support themselves. In turn, they later support their elderly parents. These obligations are based on a sense of honor that often transcends economic considerations.[4] Parents, for instance, accept their children continuing to live with them if they cannot afford their own premises. After moving out of their parents' homes the most crucial support children are supposed to give is financial. However, support can take many forms. Regular visiting and participating in social occasions of significance for the parents are also important. The family life cycle is completed when children find jobs with incomes large enough to establish separate households. Failure to do so forces children back to their parents, who sometimes have to host children and grandchildren.

As I mentioned in the introduction to my study, my first contact with the families started by developing one close relationship with a man called Sultan and his family. Sultan, who is forty years old, was born and raised in *Būlāq*. Eleven years before our meeting he married Shahira and moved in with her family, which is composed of her parents and seven siblings. My relations with Sultan and the other members of his wife's family, known in the neighborhood by the name of their father, Abu Hassan, assisted me in developing other relations with the nine other families who form the sample for this chapter.

Table 2.1 summarizes the composition of the household and dwelling spaces. I divide the ten households into three groups. The first group consists of extended families (A, B, and C). The second group (D) and (E) consists of two nuclear families. The last group includes five households that are

Table 2.1. Household Composition and Dwelling Spaces Available

Household	*Household Members*	*No. of Rooms*	*Household Composition*
			Extended Families
A	11	5	Husband and wife Three sons and one daughter A married daughter with husband and one son A widowed daughter with one son
B	9	2	Husband and wife Three sons and three daughters Wife's mother
C	6	3	Husband and wife Three sons and one daughter
			Nuclear Families
D	4	3	Husband and wife One daughter and one son
E	4	4	Husband and wife One daughter and one son
			Remnant Families
F	3	2	A widow Two daughters
G	3	3	A widow Two daughters
H	2	3	A widow One daughter
I	1	1	A widow
J	1	3	A widow
Totals	**44**	**29**	

headed by widows.[5] They are the smallest in size and the least complex in structure. A closer look at the family structures and life cycles of households reveal complexities that the general types do not represent. After I discuss the general characteristics of people living in these households, I will focus on households (A), (D), and (E) to discuss different aspects of family and individual life in *Būlāq*.

As shown in table 2.1, nine of the families live in places composed of more than one room. One lives in a single room. All of them pay low rents under government control. Rents in *Būlāq* are very low compared to other, newer, quarters of the city where prices are subject to market forces. These higher rents, and other conditions, such as unemployment, have prevented many adult members of the families from moving out. This constraint results in crowding, which is a source of constant complaint for every single individual in the three households (A, B, and C). Family members resort to a variety of short-term solutions to overcome this problem. One daughter from household (A) often spends days at a female friend's house a few streets away. On days when she returns from work and the friend is not available, she spends some hours at the mosque located on the way. During the daytime, she says there is no personal space in the house. A very similar situation exists in the second and third households. The second has two bedrooms for nine members, a small space in the middle for sitting, a kitchen, and a bathroom. Seven people actually live permanently in the house. These are the husband and the wife, their three daughters and son, and the wife's mother. The other two are sons who work as wage laborers. They keep moving between their parents' and other friends' houses. Sometimes they come home late at night just to sleep and leave next morning. The two bedrooms in this house are for the husband and the wife and the other for the wife's mother. The other room in the middle is used by all the members for eating, sitting, and, sometimes, sleeping. The third household (C) has six members, although originally it had two more sons who moved away to other neighboring quarters after they married. I include this household in the extended category because the sons and daughter are grown up and have been in marriages with children produced although they were not present in the household at the time of my study.

Other social and economic characteristics of all the households are summarized in tables 2.2 and 2.3. As shown in table 2.2, more than half (23, 52 percent) of the study group is between twenty and fifty years old,

Table 2.2. Household Age Structure

Household	*1–20 Years of Age*	*20–50 Years of Age*	*50–70 Years of Age*	*Total*
A	2	7	2	**11**
B	4	3	2	**9**
C	1	3	2	**6**
D	2	2	—	**4**
E	—	3	1	**4**
F	—	2	1	**3**
G	1	2	—	**3**
H	—	1	1	**2**
I	—	—	1	**1**
J	—	—	1	**1**
Total	**10**	**23**	**11**	**44**

Households by age and number of people.

Table 2.3. Social and Economic Characteristics of the Study Group

	Sex		*Marital Status*			*Education*				*Employment*				
Household	*M*	*F*	*Sg*	*Md*	*Wd*	*Ud*	*Dip*	*Rw*	*I*	*Hw*	*Emp*	*Rt*	*Ue*	*Total*
A	7	4	6	4	1	0	1	10	0	1	6	2	2	11
B	4	5	6	2	1	0	0	2	7	1	1	1	6	9
C	4	2	4	2	0	1	0	4	1	1	2	0	3	6
D	2	2	2	2	0	0	1	2	1	1	1	0	2	4
E	2	2	2	2	0	0	2	2	0	1	1	0	2	4
F	0	3	2	0	1	0	1	1	1	1	1	0	1	3
G	0	3	2	0	1	0	1	1	1	1	2	0	0	3
H	0	2	1	0	1	0	1	1	0	1	0	0	1	2
I	0	1	0	0	1	0	0	1	0	0	0	0	1	1
J	0	1	0	0	1	0	0	0	1	0	0	0	1	1
Total	**20**	**24**	**25**	**12**	**7**	**1**	**7**	**24**	**12**	**8**	**14**	**3**	**19**	
Total	**44**		**44**			**44**				**44**				**44**

Key
Marital status: Sg = Single, **Md** = married, **Wd** = Widowed
Education: Ud = University degree, **Dip** = Diploma, **Rw** = Read and Write, **I** = Illiterate
Employment: Hw = Housewife, **Emp** = Employed, **Rt** = Retired, **Ue** = Unemployed

a quarter (11, 25 percent) between one and twenty years, and ten or 22 percent between fifty and seventy years old. Table 2.2 summarizes another set of characteristics including sex, marital status, education, and employment. Education and employment have special meaning here. The majority of the persons can read and write. Some family members received adult education; others learned in primary and preparatory schools or obtained diplomas. "Diploma" in Egypt means study for two years after preparatory school. It is given to those who do not pass their high school entrance examination. A diploma offers several streams of knowledge and practical training, including commerce, accounting, and training for metal and woodwork. The government sponsors education in Egypt and the cost is kept relatively low. Nevertheless, not many people can remain in school because their families need them to work and contribute to the income of the domestic unit.

As for employment, I use the term "employed" to mean those who generate or receive incomes. In general terms, in *Būlāq* individuals are expected to generate incomes between the ages of twenty and fifty. In table 2.3 there are twenty-three of these people. In table 2.3 seventeen people generate incomes (fourteen working and three retired and receiving a pension). There are eight housewives. The remaining two are widowed and do not consider themselves housewives. There are nineteen unemployed. All this has great importance for the way people pool their resources and enter into long-term deals in which they depend on one another during times of hardship. As such, families represent an economic center for members who are expected to work on their separate life trajectory and save money to support themselves in the future.

Table 2.4 summarizes employment in relation to gender composition of the study group. The seventeen people who generate incomes are eleven men and six women. A closer look at the employed men and women gives a picture that is different from the one that is officially recognized especially with regard to men. Not all the men who generate incomes are actually permanently employed. Only three of them have stable or permanent jobs. The remaining five are hired for the short term by different workshops in *Būlāq* to do jobs such as repairing household items, welding, moving furniture, installing electrical circuits, painting houses, etcetera. They are paid for their labor after they finish their assignments. These men represent a large group of people in *Būlāq*. They are known as *arzaqiyya* or day-to-day bread earners. Their incomes are very significant in the survival of their families because the amount of money they earn is occasionally higher than that which is earned by government employees, such as the women who are all permanently employed for fixed salaries of no more than 150 Egyptian pounds a month. Their jobs, however, carry benefits such as health insurance and pension schemes.

Table 2.4. Gender and Employment

		Employed		*Retired*		*Unemployed*		
Household	*Housewife*	*M*	*F*	*M*	*F*	*M*	*F*	*Total*
A	1	3	3	2	0	2	0	**11**
B	1	1	0	1	0	2	4	**9**
C	1	2	0	0	0	2	1	**6**
D	1	1	0	0	0	1	1	**4**
E	1	1	0	0	0	1	1	**4**
F	1	0	1	0	0	0	1	**3**
G	1	0	2	0	0	0	0	**3**
H	1	0	0	0	0	0	1	**2**
I	0	0	0	0	0	0	1	**1**
J	0	0	0	0	0	0	1	**1**
Total	8	8	6	3	0	8	1	**4**
Total	8	14		3		19		**4**

The nature of the jobs of the *arzaqiyya* requires men to have several skills because they are always having to switch from one set of skills to another depending on the opportunity offered. Many, too, have to pretend that they can do certain jobs that often arouse suspicion about their competence. The term *fahlawi* (which best translates as "savvy" or "nimble" or to a lesser extent as "streetwise") refers to a person who is, or is seen to be, able to do difficult jobs. As the unemployed, these men have no help from the government, material or otherwise, a condition that keeps their life circumstances highly uncertain and many of their dreams and plans unfulfilled. A large number remain single until after the age of thirty-five, which is far beyond the preferred marrying age.

Now, I focus on the life in households (A), (D), and (E), where a network between the three units illustrates many aspects of family life in *Būlāq*, including the family life cycle and the use of space along lines of gender, age, and position in the household structure. These three households contain people from three generations. Figure 2.1 illustrates their genealogy. The oldest generation consists of the original parents, Abu Hassan (seventy years) and Um Hassan (sixty years). The couple moved to the neighborhood from al-Darb al-Ahmar in Old Cairo forty-five years ago.

The second generation is composed of their eight children. Two children, the oldest daughter Hassanat (forty-eight years) and the next younger son, Hassan (forty-five years), are married to partners from their age group and from the same neighborhood. Hassanat was married at the age of fifteen and

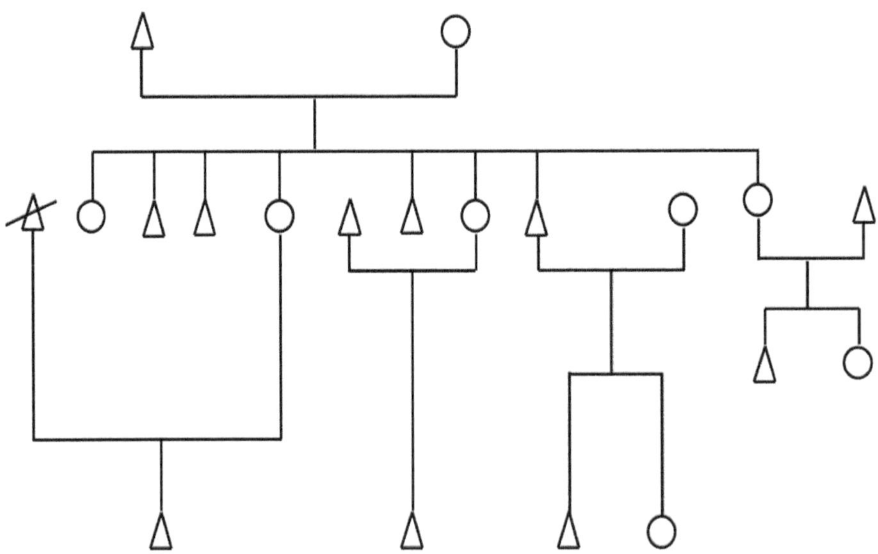

Figure 2.1. Genealogy of Hag Abu Hassan's Family

Hassan in his early twenties. They moved to live with their spouses in separate apartments. Now Hassanat has one son, Essaam (twenty-five years) and one daughter, Mervet (twenty years). Likewise, Hassan has one son, Tamir (fifteen years) and one daughter, Nirmeen (twenty-one years).

The other six children are Shahira (forty-two years), Nasser (forty years), Salwa (thirty-eight years), Khaldun (thirty-five years), and the twins Sherif (twenty-six years) and Amal (twenty-seven years). They are still living with their parents. Except for Shahira and Salwa none have ever married. Shahira was married ten years ago and her husband moved to live in her parents' apartment where they had their only son, Faady (eight years). Salwa was married twelve years ago and moved out to live with her husband. She had one son, Waael who is now eleven years old. Five years after her marriage her husband died in an accident and she returned to live with her parents.[6] Her deceased husband's family wanted to use her room for their other son who was getting married.

Abu Hassan's two eldest children had no problem finding new houses upon their marriages. Their younger siblings could not afford that. Both men and women in Cairo are required to contribute to starting their marital home. In general terms, men are expected to be married in their mid-twenties. Women are supposed to be married around the age of twenty, which is older than the age at which Hassanat was married. Before marriage, both partners have to work and save money. Men are supposed to provide the down payment to rent the apartment, pay a dowry, and buy new clothes for their brides. Women have to provide a trousseau (*gihāz*) of furniture and accoutrements and cover the costs of the wedding party. Families often prepare their daughters for marriage by buying or helping them to afford their *gihāz*. In contrast, men are expected to be the main providers of the money required to finance marital life.

Abu Hassan's sons have never had stable jobs, while the daughters have always been in employment. Salwa and Amal work for the Ministry of Religious Endowments and Shahira works as a housekeeper. Employed or not, none of these children has so far been able to save the money to move out. The result is that they have to live in a home perceived as less than adequate for their number. I was used to hearing Um Hassan's cynical, if not bitter remark: I cannot remember when this house was turned into wards (*'Anaabir*)! *'Anābir* (singular *'Anbar*) refers to different sections in hospitals or public shelters.

Figure 2.2 illustrates the living arrangements in the home of Abu Hassan's family. The area is slightly less than 100 square meters. The apartment is the top floor of a six-story building. Entering the house through the building's poorly maintained stairs (no. 1) leads to the living room (no. 2) that also leads

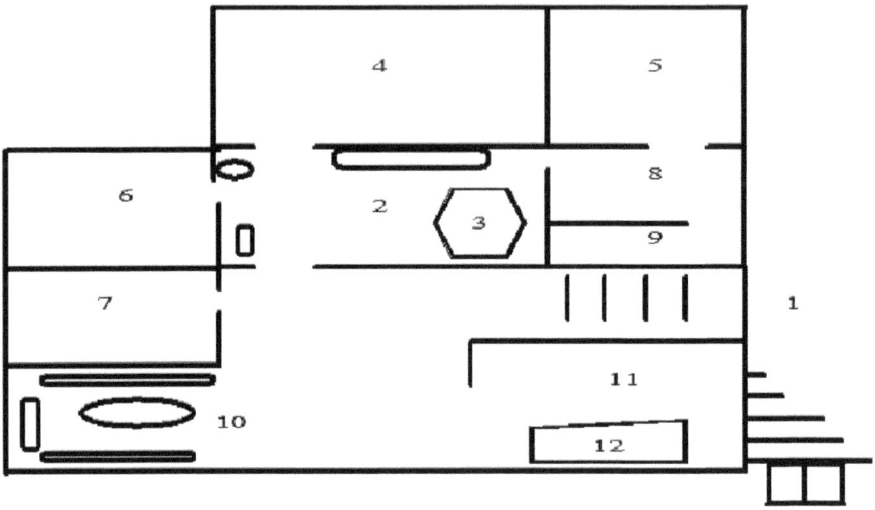

Figure 2.2. Hag Abu Hassan's House
Key:

1. Door and stairs of the building
2. Living room and passageway
3. TV set
4. Bedroom for Hag Abu Hassan and his wife
5. Bedroom for Shami, Shadya, and their eight-year-old son Karim
6. Bedroom for two daughters; one is a widow with an eleven-year-old son
7. Bedroom for three of the sons
8. Kitchen, stove, refrigerator
9. Shower room and toilet
10. Open air sitting space
11. Laundry and storage space
12. Chicken coop

to the kitchen and the bathroom shared by the whole family. The living room is the place where all the members sit to eat and to watch TV (no. 3). This is the center of the family's collective life. The TV, which is usually turned on for most of the day and night, is a constant source of entertainment and information. Alternatively, the family often sits on the roof of the apartment below them. This was turned into a balcony-like structure (no. 10) after the sons built a fence edging it. This space, referred to as *ḥawsh*, or courtyard, brings cool, fresh air during summer evenings. It also provides a space to do the laundry to which all the members contribute by using a half-automatic washing machine stationed there (no. 11). The *ḥawsh* is also an open space where males sit and play cards, and the family holds big dinners or occasional parties. In the corner of the *ḥawsh* the family once placed a little chicken coop (no. 12), hoping it would provide commodities that are otherwise too expensive. From the *ḥawsh* of Abu Hassan's house, I could see several other *aḥwāsh* with similar arrangements. Some housed goats and ducks.

The use of space in Abu Hassan's house is designated according to certain cultural rules that have been adjusted to the family's circumstances. The rules require spouses to share the same bedrooms, to place children in separate rooms in the first or second year after birth, and to separate sisters and brothers at an age well before puberty. After puberty each individual is supposed to have at least a separate spot for sleeping. Looking at the family's sleeping arrangements shows that the rules are applied only in the case of Abu Hassan and his wife, who have a separate bedroom (no. 4) for themselves. This privilege is not extended to Sultan and his wife, who have to share their bedroom (no. 5) with their eight-year-old son. Likewise, Salwa has to share her bedroom (no. 6) with her sister Amal, and her bed with her eleven-year-old son Waael. The three sons have to share one small bedroom (no. 7) where two of them sleep in one bed. The arrangement obviously accords with cultural rules, but only up to a point because of the shortage of space.

In these circumstances, stability is impossible without the family members' established sense of sharing, tolerance, and sacrifice. In *Būlāq* there is a common saying which expresses this idea and which was repeated by Abu Hassan many times: *guhri l-dīb yusa' mit ḥabīb* (even a hole for a wolf can take a hundred friends, or lovers). Of course, this optimism does not rule out conflict over limited resources, including space. Conflict deriving from living in adverse material circumstances engenders anger and dissatisfaction (*za'al*), which are often given as primary sources of illness—as discussed in chapter 3.

The families of the oldest daughter Hassanat (E) and son Hassan (D) live in very different conditions and show arrangements in line with the cultural criteria their unmarried siblings cannot fulfill. Hassanat has been married for the last thirty years and lives in a separate house (E) with her husband, son, and daughter. She moved to her husband's house upon marrying and is currently almost totally independent of her parents. Her living arrangements allow her a separate room for herself and her husband and a room for each of her children. Similarly, Hassan has his own apartment where space is allocated to give privacy to him and his wife, and each of his two children.

Hassanat and Hassan obviously have nuclear families with a less complex structure than that of their parents' household. However, both nuclear families might enlarge if the children stay after their marriages. In contrast to their parents, both families chose to have fewer children. They were aware that younger generations would have to face problems such as those experienced by Abu Hassan's other children who could not afford marriage and apartments in a market characterized by rapid inflation and a diminished number of jobs. Hassan and Hassanat also suffer from similar problems by worrying about the future life of their children who, at some point, will face conditions similar to those experienced by their younger brothers. As such, individuals in *Būlāq* are hard to distinguish as separate agents away from their families. Their incomes, which are perceived as lower than their needs, coupled with the rising cost of living, make their economic life highly uncertain and their family ties an indispensable means for managing various life circumstances, including health problems. Family members are always engaged in long-term transactions with each other based on relations of kinship and friendship.

HEALTH EXPERIENCE

Many daily incidents taught me the rampant nature of illness in *Būlāq*. Of the fifty-seven persons with whom I conducted interviews, thirty-three had at least one health complaint for which they had sought help. This prevalence of illness makes issues of health and therapy a constantly communicated theme of everyday life: different disease therapies are compared and evaluated. Illness is not viewed as isolated from people's family lives and obligations; the physical body is perceived as an extension of an affectionate and intimate social life. In the next section, I will discuss these narratives in relation to the different ways the individual can be perceived in connection to family life and the social body.

Sharing Medical Knowledge

The following situation illustrates how health is perceived in terms of relations between individuals rather than as a property of the individual *per se*. Secondly, it shows how medical knowledge is routinely exchanged between relatives. Thirdly, it demonstrates how therapies are pragmatically combined. They are viewed as different but complementary means of ensuring healing.

It is Friday noon in *Būlāq* and the quarter is quiet. The surrounding workshops and markets are closed. Some men are walking toward mosques for prayers. Other men sit and smoke water pipes (*shīsha*), drink tea, and talk over a whole variety of issues and concerns. Wives are at home taking care of the children and preparing a meal for the family. I am spending this Friday with Abu Hassan's family. On the unpaved alley that leads to the building where the family lives, I notice Sultan sitting in a café. I walk up to him and join him at his little table. Sultan is sitting with Hassan, his eldest brother-in-law. After exchanging greetings with other men, I join Sultan at his table. As we exchanged greetings I included the common question: *izzayṣṣiḥḥah?*—how is the (meaning your) health doing? Hassan looks very concerned. He replies,

> It is too bad, pupils at the school think my son is *magnū* (possessed or mad). You know, when he does not take the pill (*'il-birshām*), he cannot walk in a straight line. He walks like a drunken man. It kills me when I remember that he got that damn germ thing at the hospital. He went there to be treated for a cough. He spent few days there but came out with this disaster.

What is of overwhelming importance here is the manner in which a question concerning Hassan's own health automatically becomes a question of his son's health. Hassan's fifteen-year-old son, Tamir, suffers from the consequences of an infection he caught shortly after spending a few days in the nearby public hospital two years ago. His relatives know that he has to carry on taking specific, and thus expensive, medicines in order to help him cope with nerve (*'a'ṣāb*) problems resulting from the infection. Everybody knows about Tamir's problem. Hassan wants to share his desperation and perhaps seek suggestions or information gathered by others. I know that he has been trying an endless number of solutions, including going to expensive clinics and a number of herb shops in the neighborhood and beyond.

Hassan is the only breadwinner for his four-member family. In addition to Tamir, Hassan lives with his forty-year-old wife, Nuha, and twenty-one-year-old daughter, Nirmeen. The family is completely dependent on his income, which comes from painting and decorating houses. From this income Hassan also has to provide medicine for his wife. For the last few years she has been suffering from back pain. The conditions of his wife and son lead to considerable expense, limiting the financial prospects of the family. They seem to have no solution. This is perhaps why Sultan commented sympathetically: "*rabbina yishfih ya rāgil* (may God cure him, man), what else could one say? That is his share in life, you never know what disasters could happen these days." Then, as a means of sharing suffering as well as asking for advice, Sultan directs attention to his own problem: "You know, I even cannot deal with these boils on my lips. They are too painful, I don't know how they come." Although immersed in his thoughts about his son and wife, Hassan promptly replies: "Listen, it is very easy, just go to that pharmacy down the street. They are open on Friday. Get some *muḍāḍ* (antibiotic) . . . any kind can help. Then, go to the bakery next door and get some *khimīrah* (yeast). Take *khimīrah* and the *muḍāḍ* and you will be fine in a few days." Sultan follows Hassan's advice carefully, because he is understood to be knowledgeable in these matters. He has been to many places in his life. Besides traveling inside Egypt, he has worked for seven years in Jordan, Syria, and Iraq. He always looks confident when talking to the other family members, who listen and often follow his advice. I ask Sultan how yeast can cure boils. He is determined to explain Hassan's authoritative advice,

> The yeast can take care of my stomach, which now must be very hot and dry. It is just some heat in the stomach but it shows on the lips. The yeast can cool it down. The antibiotics can kill the germs that must be somewhere and caused the boils.

This encounter shows how the activity of consoling is also a way of exchanging information about health between family members and friends. It is through this activity that multiple therapies are suggested and discussed. It also shows how multiple therapies are used simultaneously to cure different aspects of disease.

Life Presses On My Soul

In terms of therapy, an individual body is not produced simply as a function of theories of treatment. On the way to the body, these theories are evaluated and adjusted in light of family ties and material circumstances and constraints. Secondly, the borderline between "physical" ill health and other pains cannot be clearly drawn. Illness is not only a somatic problem. It is seen in terms of the soul, or *al-nafs*, which can manifest itself physically. Knowledge used to treat illness therefore is multiple. They all interact to form a unified notion of being that has to do not only with the individual self, but also with that self defined in relation to the social body including the family and larger networks.

Shahira is forty-two years old. She has been married to Sultan for the last ten years. She works as a housekeeper for a social club within a boathouse on the Nile. Shahira looks much happier at work than she does at home. She feels that her house is too crowded and noisy. In addition to her pride at working outside the house, she also talks freely about her unhappiness with her husband who has been on a pension for several years and sits at home most of the day. At the same time, he expects her to do the housework. Shahira had to find a job to make up for her husband's small income. Her salary of 100 Egyptian pounds plus her husband's pension of 150 Egyptian pounds are used to support herself, her husband, and their son. This small family pays a small share to Shahira's mother who manages the whole of Abu Hassan's house. Every day Shahira works at the boathouse, takes care of her son, and contributes to the housework of her larger family. Shahira was illiterate but has started going to adult education evening classes administered by a government school in *Būlāq*.

For the last four years Shahira has been suffering from a pain in her lower back on the right-hand side. This pain is very common among lower class families in Cairo and is generally said to be caused by kidney problems. It is referred to as *waga' ganb* (body side pain). When she felt the pain for the first time, Shahira went with her husband to a general practitioner in the neighborhood. The practitioner prescribed analgesics (*musakkimāt*)[7] and sent her for laboratory tests. She bought the medicines and had the tests, but could not afford the second visit to the doctor. She had already spent the whole fifty Egyptian pounds set aside over several months on her son who had broken his arm. For the last four years she has lived with this occasional pain and in the hope she will recover.

Shahira's pain has a particular meaning for her that relates to her living conditions, her family, and her perception of her position in society. In her attempts to answer the question "why did this pain happen to me?" Shahira shifts between three explanations. First and foremost she refers to her "lot in life" (*naṣib*), related to having less money than she wishes and having to put up with a man who is unable to support her. Shahira refers to these conditions in times of desperation and sometimes during fights with other family members. On such occasions she mentions the word *il-ghulb*, meaning "the defeat," as an overall explanation of her lot in life. She does not mean that misfortune can explain her illness; misfortune has to do with the material conditions since she was born. The concept of *il-ghulb* implies that she has been trying, and even fighting, to improve matters.

In dealing with aspects of her illness, Shahira has specific ways of thinking and acting. At some points, she refers to "cold" as the main cause of her illness. At others, she refers to the possibility of a stone or a germ in her kidney that causes the pain. Although different, these two causes are seen as interrelated. Whether it is cold, a stone, or a germ, Shahira thinks that keeping her body warm stops, or at least reduces, the pain. She states confidently that the pain occurs because of increased dampness: "I used to leave my body wet for hours after showers." As a way of coping with the pain she says she tries to keep warm and dry. Sometimes, however, she takes a more biomedical view and wonders whether a solution lies there: but she is aware that it is more difficult to afford. I met Shahira in pain several times, walking back home with her right hand on her back. When she has no access to painkillers, which she knows she can buy from pharmacies, she suffers for a day or two.

Shahira's experience in health and illness is shaped by a physician's advice, her mother's opinions, sisters' and brothers' ideas, and neighbors' suggestions, as well as her own experiments. At home, her mother's guidance concerning how to treat common illnesses is an important source of her health knowledge. Many times, I saw Shahira's mother commenting on the advice and therapies her children had received from physicians. Being illiterate,

Shahira does not use pamphlets or books to guide her methods of healing. However, she often watches TV programs about health and medicine. She also follows advice from friends who can read written sources.

Shahira's illness takes on an additional dimension when situated in her family life. Shahira's husband does not work. He is retired because he has *daran*, an old infection in his lungs that has weakened his breathing capacity. His pension is too small to cover his family's living costs. At times he takes money from his brother who works abroad. However, Shahira always expresses her extreme unhappiness at their living arrangements. They are living in one room and have to share the kitchen, bathroom, and living room with other members of the household. Shahira's honor is injured because her husband does not provide her with housing and this makes her feel unequal to other women. When she married she had hoped he would soon find something better.

Shahira's life conditions and health status are closely connected to those of her only son, Faady. A few months ago Faady was playing with other children when he fell and broke his arm. At the nearest public hospital where his father took him, a doctor on duty decided that the arm was fractured and needed plaster. The cost was fifty Egyptian pounds, which the father could not provide. Meanwhile, Shahira had some money that she had collected for her next visit to a physician. She had to pay that money for the materials necessary to set her son's arm. Beginning to cry, she bitterly says,

> it is the arm of my son; he is all that I have got in this life. He will be a grown man and he will need healthy arms to earn his bread and be a respectable person, I want him to receive the best opportunities in life and to be whatever he wishes to be.

Ironically, a few months later, Shahira had saved some more money and wanted to go to the doctor. Then again, her son broke his same arm. This time, she even had to borrow money over and above what she had.

All these conditions "press down my soul" Shahira says sadly. Every once in a while, while talking to me, she would say with a deep sigh: "it is not going well, but at least it is going." This ambivalence about her life conditions makes her look as though she is ready to explode with anger and to speak violently about other people including her co-workers and, at times, other family members.

On Child's Health

Faady's case illustrates the way the family is connected to a larger network of friends and neighbors. After the second accident, Faady's father thought that the arm was broken and immediately took him to the nearby public hospital.

The child was examined by the doctor on duty, who decided that there was no serious problem. The father believed him and returned home with the child. At home, Faady kept complaining of a persistent pain in his arm. A few hours later, his father took him to a private hospital, which was possible as Faady has school health insurance. At the private hospital the father luckily found a friend of the family working as a physician.

The doctor told the father to feed Faady milk and other rich food such as eggs and take him back to the hospital after thirty-two days. At that prearranged time I accompanied the father and his child. Khaldun, Shahira's brother, also came along. At the hospital two X-rays were taken of the affected arm and the doctor recommended that the cast should stay on for two more weeks. After two weeks the father took his son back to the hospital where they removed the plaster. The arm was obviously not as straight as it should have been. The father asked why, to which the doctor replied: "It is because the arm was broken twice. The child is still young and his arm will grow straight. The crooked part will disappear when the arm grows bigger."

I did not think the doctor's explanation would be accepted but Faady's father looked convinced. At home, family members were upset about the outcome of the treatment. However, within a few days they seemed to have accepted it because they could not afford further treatment. Acceptance of the advice of the doctor was not smooth though. Sayyid, Abu Hassan's sixty-year-old friend of many years' standing who lives nearby, suggested that they should return to the hospital so that the arm could be broken again and reset. The father rejected the idea because it would be too difficult for his young son and too expensive. Members of the family were unsure whether further treatment would be better than the first time. On the surface they all accepted the outcome, but none of them expressed satisfaction. Between feelings of disappointment about the hospital's bad treatment, uncertainty over other options, inability to cover the higher costs for further therapy, family members did not accept or reject the therapy, but rather saw the treatment in a pragmatic light that kept the door open for future solutions.

PERCEIVED SOCIAL DISTRESS: "WE HAVE ACCEPTED DISTRESS, BUT IT NEVER ACCEPTED US"

The following family case gives a new perspective on health and the social origins of illness. Instead of speaking about life in abstract terms, the main characters conceptualize living conditions within social transformations taking place beyond family boundaries. Sultan's eldest sister-in-law, Hassanat, is a forty-eight-year-old woman who lives with her husband, son, and daughter. Their house is located many blocks away from her parents.

Hassanat says she is a "*sitti bait*" (a house lady), as housewives are referred to in Cairo. However, in her case this is not completely accurate: it is rather what she hopes for. Her husband, Hag Ahmed, has a little candy store down the street a few meters from their apartment. In addition to her work at home, she runs the store with him. I first met the family at their shop and later at their home as the relationship grew friendlier and more informal.

Most of my discussions with them centered around the family's life and their daily circumstances. Hassanat and Ahmed married twenty-five years ago, and were determined to break with their parents' way of life. First of all this meant having fewer children. Hassanat used contraceptive pills, but after a short time she stopped taking the pills because she felt they had a bad affect on her health. A month later she became pregnant. She bore Essaam, her son, and after his birth she started taking the pill again, which she did for the next five years. Subsequently, she "wished Essaam to have a brother or a sister," and she had Mervet, her daughter.

The couple, proud to be called Um and Abu Essaam (mother and father of Essaam), agree it was the mother who insisted on not having more than two children. She says:

> I am the one who suffers during pregnancy and giving birth. I suffered from living in a large family: actually, as the eldest I was the one who raised my sisters and brothers. I also wanted to give my children the best, and the opportunity to have whatever they ask for. I wanted them to have a good education and good jobs so that they could get married to people from good families (*awlād nās*).

After having the daughter, Um Essaam was sterilized. As the quotation suggests, her decision not to have children is tied to her experience in her family. She complains that after the sixth grade her mother forced her out of school in order to help raise her younger brothers and sisters and assist with the housework. Although she was not introduced to contraception through formal education, Um Essaam was aware of the importance of controlling her fertility. It is obvious that her children have a better lifestyle and are better dressed than most children in the neighborhood. Both children have finished high school and have higher diplomas.

Having college degrees only triggers a new stage in Um Essaam's concern about her children. They have to succeed and find jobs. When I first met the family their daughter, Mervet, was sitting for her final college examinations. Her chances of passing were a constant source of worry. When she passed, the family, including Um Essaam's mother, brothers and sisters and their children, jointly celebrated her success. Furthermore, during my research,

Essaam started a small advertising company, investing his savings in the project. His chances of success were also a constant topic of family discussion.

The family has a very smooth cooperative domestic life: The parents were the only couple in the study that spoke of their affectionate relationship and how it had continued over the years. Throughout their married life, however, the couple has suffered from a variety of illnesses. However, unlike Shahira, Um and Abu Essaam emphasize the economic difficulties they encountered as external factors. They both believe that those hardships somehow engendered their bodily pains. Um Essaam complains of heart problems, an inflamed gall bladder, and pain in her right knee. In addition, she occasionally has headaches that come "when I do excessive amounts of work," as she puts it. Um Essaam uses the names of diseases mentioned by doctors. Nevertheless, she thinks that her health problems are not purely physical, although they may appear so,

> they originally have to do with my soul (*ḥālah nafsiyya*). This demanding life and pressing economic needs can produce a lot of imbalance in my *nafs* (soul). High prices can cause tension because I cannot find proper solutions or answers for my problems and questions. Hopelessness leads to despair, which can make me very tired and unhappy about myself.

After a reflective pause,

> it is the way life has been going downhill for the several years that gives me all these pains. My family is a very happy one. My husband is an understanding person and a very warm and supportive man. My children are successful and they do what I say (*biysma'u ilkilmah*). The problem is not my family; it is the world around us . . . pressures from life are increasing.

Then, pointing to her earlier aspirations for a better life,

> We cannot manage to live in the way society requires us to do. It [the cost of living] was very low in the past, but then the prices rose. We said OK, and bowed to the storm (*waṭaina rasna li al-'aṣifah*). We accepted the challenge and wanted to go on. We understood that we should adapt, and thought things would get better soon. But things continued going downhill, and now they are not going well. It feels as though we accepted distress, but it never accepted us (*ridina bilham, bassi l-ham mardish bīna*).

An important reason for Um Essaam's state of distress is uncertainty about her children's futures, which causes great anxiety for her and her husband. Religion has been one way to cope with the uncertainty in their life. Um Essaam finds relief only in her belief that God will eventually provide an unexpected solution. She recently became more observant about religion and started to wear longer dresses and a headscarf. Her husband also started to pray more regularly in the mosque a few steps from his shop.

For the last three years Abu Essaam has been suffering from numbness in his left arm. A doctor in a private clinic told him that his pain was the result of a dislocated vertebra pressing on a nerve. Abu Essaam has gathered a lot of information on his condition during his conversations with many people, including various physicians. However, none of the explanations totally satisfies him. He always felt some bad spirit "touched" him and that this was the cause of his illness. Both Abu Essaam and his wife suggested this cause. Once he described how a saint (*wali*) touched him when passing the shop, and how wonderful he felt for the next few days. Abu Essaam believes the *wali's* touch could have healed him had he followed and found him again. Like Shahira, at points Abu Essaam would switch between different explanatory methods. He also mentioned that his illness might have been caused by him having stopped smoking hashish several years ago: "it has become terribly expensive and so difficult to get," he says. As in the previous cases, multiple explanations are at work here.

As I discussed different issues with the couple, we inevitably ended up speaking about their economic crisis, the corrupt government, and the lack of employment that diminished their children's opportunities. Abu and Um Essaam are aware that these conditions affect the whole country. They started to feel the worsening economic crisis in the country in the late 1980s when the prices of goods rose dramatically and job opportunities grew scarce. The rising cost of living was associated with news about corruption in the government. Um Essaam and Abu Essaam think that the chronic economic crisis, which started in the mid-1980s, affected them when members of their economic class split between those who could move to the upper classes and those who were forced to go down on the socioeconomic ladder. More people went down than up. Fear of further descent always features in the family's conversations.

CONCLUSION

So far I have introduced the history and present life setting of *Būlāq*, including the available medical resources. I also described a group of households connected through a network based on kinship and friendship. Finally, I presented a group of narratives about the recent health experiences of three families. The history of *Būlāq* illustrates that several elements from the past continue to influence the individuals' health practices: there are multiple health resources, primarily modern medicine, herb-based therapies, and spiritual healing.

The family occupies a pivotal role in organizing the lives of individuals who rely on its advice about their health problems. However, the family can also be seen as a source of ill health because of the tensions, demands, and obligations it engenders. This sets up a complex pattern of interaction. First, individuals constantly explain their physical pain in terms of family problems. They include their emotions as quintessential elements of their experience of pain.

Second, the decisions and actions of the individuals stem from their family structures. The scene of the men sitting at the café discussing health and other issues, and the whole family of Abu Hassan becoming involved in the problem of their grandson's broken arm, illustrate how families collaborate and pass on information about health and illness. The discussion of Shahira's illness shows how several therapeutic methods can be employed and also how the procedures she chooses are intrinsically connected to her son and husband. In practice, Shahira's health and body are products of her social relations.

Third, people use multiple therapies, including biomedicine, herbal therapies, and spiritual healing. They value biomedicine very highly, but they do not consider it as *essentially* different from herb-based medicines, or as incompatible with spiritual healing. The therapies derived from all these sources are sometimes used simultaneously. The herbs are viewed as the predecessors of biochemical medicines. Spiritual healing complements other forms of therapy because it is concerned with bringing the sick body, as an imbalanced state of being, back to harmonious normality.

Fourth, connected to the above points and central to explaining the process of falling ill is the notion of *al-nafs*, which in Arabic refers to both the modern concept of the *al-'aql* (the "mind") contrasted to *al-jasad* (the "body"), and to a popular older concept that combines the body and the mind. From the latter point of view, the notion of *al-nafs* refers to a completely integrated state of being that reflects well-being in both physical and spiritual terms. It is the space where both the mind and the body are fused: the mind is embodied and the body is spirited.

This pattern of behavior is different from the world of health and medicine as constituted in professional settings where the patient's social life and values and moral attitudes are not normally part of the medical evaluation/examination. The lives of the individuals are constituted as a medical problem based on a series of dichotomies that represent the deep cultural logic of the dominant biomedical discourse. The narratives bring elements different from biomedicine that assumes that individuals are sovereign agents, or as distinct entities prior to society and culture. It is best to envisage individuals in this study as *networked* or rather *reticulated* agents. As such, the notion of *al-nafs* simultaneously represents individuals and their consciousness of their bodies as well as the social relations in which they live.

In conclusion, health in *Būlāq* is shaped by an interplay between diverse models of health care, networks of which the family is by far the most important and material practicalities. Always at issue is the social and political body, which is not an aggregate of individuals but the very means of producing and maintaining bodily identity. The centrality of this body cannot be understood using elements from one system of medical care but in the context of situations explained by notions and methods of the plural system of health care understood as one single space of interacting and changing means in continuous process of adaptation to the needs of the individuals concerned. The latter are personified by virtue of relying on the plural health resources tightly connected to family values and issues of local biology and subjectivity.

The next chapter is a focused case study of one complex cultural fact called *'iḍḍaghṭ* or "pressure." This general social complaint is constructed from elements derived from the plural medical system of Cairo. As a phenomenon, it is a cultural space where links between life conditions are mediated by emotionally mediated moral concerns. The discussion and detailed narratives of this illness will further illustrate my theory.

NOTES

1. The term *sha'biyya* is derived from the word *sha'b*, which generally means "people" or the "popular masses." Its current use points to homogeneity between various sections of society, especially in contexts of nationalism. Paradoxically, the term's root in Arabic is *sha'aba*, which literally points to differences. It means to "branch," "diversify," or "divide." Curiously, the latter meaning is most relevant in pointing to styles of living common among low-income groups of the population, which constitute the vast majority of the population. The term thus simultaneously divides and unites.

2. Population counts for individual neighborhoods in Cairo are currently inaccessible due to government regulations. I have had to resort to secondary sources in order to assess the present size of the population. The projection might not be exact; it is certainly less than the real numbers.

3. During the time of my research, 3.4 Egyptian pounds equalled $1US.

4. See Watson (1992) where she argues, based on her research in Cairo, "In Arab-Muslim society there is a complex, well-defined and highly structured set of gender roles which underpins personal and public life and gives marriage and the family a central importance" (Watson 1992: 5).

5. In Egypt, life expectancy for males is less than for females (see Rugh 1988: 182). However, the number of widows in my sample may be disproportionately large. Equally high numbers, however, have been estimated by another study of a low-income community (Kuppinger 1990: 113). This estimate suggests that low-income communities might have lower male life expectancies than other groups.

6. For a fuller account of this social rule see al-Messiri (1977: 213–214) who reports a similar social context where the rule of returning to the parents' home applies to men and women after the death of a spouse. If the parents are deceased, the divorcee or widow returns to a brother, a sister, or another relative. In any case, this practice shows the continued centrality of family relations through time.

7. The word *musakkin* derives from the Arabic root *sakana,* which means to calm or tranquilize.

3

'Iḍḍaghṭ

A Biomedical Category as Cultural Critique

To further explain the ideas discussed in the previous chapter I am going to focus here on one issue in Cairo called *'iḍḍaghṭ* or pressure (pl. *ḍūghūṭ*, pressures), a hallmark of life in Cairo. Professionals of biomedicine formally link *'iḍḍaghṭ* to the well-known condition of high blood pressure or hypertension. But this is only what the biomedical gaze prepares them to see and say. It does not include what those who complain from *'iḍḍaghṭ* have to say. It also excludes those who have never tested their blood pressure and complain of *'iḍḍaghṭ*. Even more, it remains silent about others who speak about *ḍūghūṭ al-hayaah* (pressures of life) without referring to anything medical. These basic observations indicate that hypertension is not *'iḍḍaghṭ* but a different *fact* that is not biomedical but *cultural*. Today, one needs to be in Cairo for even for some days to notice that many people from different social backgrounds say that they suffer from *'iḍḍaghṭ*; it is enough to mention this word in a gathering, whether formal or informal, for a long conversation to ensue not necessary on issues directly related to health, but about politics, the soaring prices of meat and vegetables, the city's worsening pollution, overcrowding, conflict, competition, rage, and many more. This plethora of issues and problems therefore begs the question of what is it in *'iḍḍaghṭ* that calls such diverse ideas to flow all together? How could a single term be used to simultaneously describe so many complex aspects of life in Cairo? Is it the power of biomedicine or biomedicalization (Clarke 2010: 1–2) that was able to make these issues included within one term? Or was this term invented by Cairenes as a poetic emblem for their increasingly overpowering life?

I think all these and other questions find answers in Cairo's plural system of health care endowed with a multitude of resources capable of viewing life as an integrated totality. I argue that it is within this system that complex issues like *dughut al-hayaah* can best be appreciated. It is true that *'iḍḍaghṭ* is an illness felt by individuals but in Cairo these are *persons* who live with families and other groups with whom they manage their material daily life based on shared memories and future aspirations using a local language and inherited wisdom represented in this context by the multiple health resources that I think have been "Egyptianized" as it were through centuries of constant interaction and change. My argument is that *'iḍḍaghṭ* has been constructed by terms derived from these health resources combined. In this context I am concerned with the following questions. How do Cairenes define *'iḍḍaghṭ* and more importantly what do they mean whey they say they "have *'iḍḍaghṭ*"? or when they feel "tired, suffocated or disgusted by the many *ḍūghūṭ* of life?" How do they explain the occurrence of these *ḍūghūṭ*? If *'iḍḍaghṭ* is an attribute of social life, how then does it mediate to individual persons? Where do these *ḍūghūṭ* happen? How are they felt? How do they affect the individuals afflicted? What do medical professionals say about *'iḍḍaghṭ* especially when they suffer from it? How different are they from the laypersons? How is *'iḍḍaghṭ* expressed, especially when there are no symptoms recognized?

In brief, this chapter is concerned with *'iḍḍaghṭ* as a cultural construction and its implications for the social relations of power. Analytically, health care practices occur in accordance to social formations that decide the society's ways of life. Egypt has been developed into a globalized peripheral capitalist society. *Dughut al-hayaah* so rampant in Cairo according to the participants in this research as well as official reports must have been generated by the country's changed socioeconomic relations which were shifted to neoliberal economics starting in the late 1970s. The product has so far been crony capitalism. Meanwhile, the market experienced soaring prices, high rates of inflation, and expanding consumer culture associated with great expansion of the commercial media. The latter exacerbated the distance between people's material capacities on the one hand and their enhanced desires for consumption. In such context a small proportion of the population coming from different economic backgrounds managed to attain high incomes either through successful investment and/or working abroad. The entire socioeconomic environment though was infested with corruption. The majority of the population experienced high rates of "poverty, unemployment, atrocious social unfairness, political oppression and maltreatment of ordinary people, which made it impossible for millions of Egyptians to live normally" (al-Aswani 2010: 10). My argument then is that radically changed economic relations were associated with inappropriate social and moral development. I think such incongruity must have perfectly corresponded to the common sense of *imbalance* sensed as excessive amounts of *'iḍḍaghṭ* as we will see in the narratives below.

I view life and health care as a single space. Cairo seems to offer one field in which one can complain about one's body pains as connected to other people, to family relations, pressures of life, and emotional pains all at once. In this context, the plural system provides multiple "discursive spaces" different from the binary constructions of biomedicine that divides states of being into two sharply separated categories of "ease" and "dis-ease" so to speak and which are not physical categories by any means. It is in fact uninteresting to speak about *'iḍḍaghṭ* as a problem caused by "physical" factors for those are essentially inseparable from the way they are articulated in the words, feelings, emotions, and ideas of those who live them. Furthermore, the plural system allows persons to express their feelings of wellness and unwellness without having to be sick as noted earlier in this study. In other words, it offers a nuanced spectrum composed of several states of being and thus allows persons to express their lives as complex shifting fields of complaints, dissatisfactions, and even indifferences.

'Iḍḍaghṭ is the Cairene shorthand term referring to high blood pressure and many other kinds of pressure believed to be inherent social, ecological, and economic conditions characterizing the city. The relationships that may exist between the condition of high blood pressure and the other conditions are not objective ones. Those who mention the two do not try to demonstrate whether those causative relationships truly exist. It is sort of a taken for granted cultural fact, or say a belief. How? Never mind, what matters is that it is mediated by negative emotions called *'izza'al* (anger) that affect the body through *al-nafs* (the soul). In this sense *'iḍḍaghṭ* is a statement to protest social conditions of living that otherwise have very small opportunity to be protested in a society experiencing excessive amounts of oppression. No single perspective can capture this kind of notion but one that aims at holism, which is an attribute of Cairo's plural system of health care.

In brief, the experience of *'iḍḍaghṭ* in Cairo be summarized as follows. It renders the body accessible through *al-nafs* and susceptible to emotions of *'izza'al* associated with suppression (*katm*). It regards individuals as persons with blurred borders with the outside world. Health is optimum balance constituted by the humors and proportions these are mixed. This health when exposed to worsening conditions characterized by declining standards of living for the middle classes and frustrated hopes for groups with lower incomes who have been encouraged to attain better lives through the media. The negative emotions of *'izza'al* lead to the construction of *'iḍḍaghṭ* to represent many states of being that while ranging between health and ill health send a message of protestation about the conditions of living as unacceptable. This construction however is not evenly distributed among different components of the plural system or between different social classes and genders. Finally, the contribution of the plural system has not been even; middle classes tended to accept and use terms offered by biomedicine while lower classes tended to accept terms offered by humoral theory. Furthermore, women mentioned *katm* more often than men.

As a whole, this chapter is divided into four sections. In the second section after this introductory note, I discuss the various definitions about *'iḍḍaghṭ* available in the press and in one self-help guide. I discuss these definitions in the context of a survey I conducted on forty patients who are identified by medical practitioners as having *'iḍḍaghṭ*. The perceptions and interpretations of these persons are presented in the contexts in which these people live, that is, their families and the city as a whole. I summarise the interpretations of *'iḍḍaghṭ* under three main headings: pressures of life, pollution, and *'izza'al*. The various ways these general categories lead to more specific causes are diagrammed in detail. Third, I present narratives of some medical practitioners who are ill with high blood pressure. The objective is to illustrate that *'iḍḍaghṭ* traverses the entire integrated field of Cairo's health resources when it is *lived* by professionals and laypersons alike. In the fourth section I include three narratives of people diagnosed with *'iḍḍaghṭ*. Finally, I discuss the theoretical implications of my findings, including the meanings of the various terms used to explain *'iḍḍaghṭ* as well as the "semantic fields" that emerge from the specific ways the social circumstances associated with *'iḍḍaghṭ* are configured in the current culture of life and health in Cairo.

The clinicians focus their "objective" gaze on this field to identify the objects to be known (Foucault 1989: x). The people who subscribe to *'iḍḍaghṭ* enter this field not for the objects it includes but for the space it provides to express the "subjective symptoms," and are often offered small, if any, opportunity to be cured. They also look in this field of opportunities to articulate their often unrecognized sense of pain into moral expressions illustrating the good plight of life so to speak; life as an opportunity of both joy and pain. My argument is that *'iḍḍaghṭ* is a complex cultural fact expressing diverse states of being characterizing life conditions in Cairo mediated through emotions. It is produced in terms offered by the city's plural medical system composed of one integrated space concerned with life as an integrated totality encompassing health as an holistic notion and not physical complaints of separate individuals. Throughout these processes of production, *'iḍḍaghṭ* speaks of social experiences, events, and situations of conflict, which are expressed in terms rooted in various traditions including primarily Greek-Islamic therapeutic methods, biochemical medicine, and other inherited wisdom. In this context the concept of hypertension is no more than one element in a larger field or social discourse organized around two main domains: the "pressures of life" (*ḍūghūṭ ḥayāh*), which I call "social pressures," and the general problem of "pollution" (*talawwuth*). These are mediated through a complex notion pointing mainly to negative emotions summed by the one term called *'izza'al*. The social pressures include the demands of the family, the living space perceived as inadequately small, as well as factors related to social inequity and political oppression. These factors are mediated by *'izza'al* (painful anger) coupled with a cultural practice of *al-katm* (suppressing the breath). The problem of pollution includes the harmful effects of the urban environment, which is perceived as responsible for producing *'iḍḍaghṭ* in addition to other endemic diseases. The pathologic effect of the contraceptive pill, which retains the blood of menstruation perceived as atrabilious, is also included under pollution.

THE SEMANTICS AND SEMIOTICS OF 'IḌḌAGHṬ

The following survey includes people from different social categories of age, social class, education, and gender. The group is composed of seventeen females and twenty-three males (table 3.1). Their ages are between twenty-six and seventy years old. Twenty-seven of them are between forty and sixty years old. They are either illiterate (thirteen people, five males and eight females) or able to read and write (nine males and five females). The remaining thirteen individuals are five (two males and three females) with high school education or diplomas and eight (seven males and one female) with university degrees (one female physician, five males with a BSc, one male with an MA and one with a PhD). This group of people consists of individuals with different social characteristics. My reason for including it is that by using it I can present more about the terms that illustrate the cultural framework within which the narratives operate. It consists of individuals with different social characteristics. The diverse social backgrounds in connection with the health status of the individuals included in the sample will reveal further dimensions of the social phenomenon of *'iḍḍaghṭ*.

Table 3.1. Age, Sex, and Education of the Individuals Included

Age			Sex		Education							
25–40	**40–60**	**60–70**	**M**	**F**	**Illiterate**		**Read and Write**		**Diploma**		**University Degree**	
6	27	7	23	17	5M	8F	9M	5F	2M	3F	7M	1F
					13		14		5		8	
40			**40**		**40**							

Table 3.2. Marital Status and Pattern of Residence

Marital Status								Pattern of Residence			
Married		Divorced		Widowed		Single		Living with Family		Living Alone	
M	F	M	F	M	F	M	F	M	F	M	F
19	9	0	1	1	7	3	0	21	14	2	3
28		1		8		3		35		5	
Total				40				40			

Most of the individuals included, twenty-nine (nineteen males and ten females), are married and live with their spouses (table 3.2), which illustrates the significance of the family for the incidence of *'iḍḍaghṭ*. All of these live or stay in close connection with their children except for three individuals who are married but have no children. Four individuals (all males) are single and six are widowed (five females and one male). Of the latter group two (one male and one female) have no children and live on their own. The rest have children who live with them. Only one female is separated from her husband while still married. Regardless of their marital status all the individuals included live in close connection with their relatives whether those be their immediate kin, sons, daughters, fathers, mothers, or some other more distant relatives. As I mentioned in the chapter on health and illness in *Būlāq* the family is a cornerstone institution in the individual's life in Cairo. In all cases it was the first and foremost reference group mentioned in individuals' interpretative and therapeutic activities. Furthermore, all the individuals mention the family and family life as a major factor contributing to their health and illness.

The complexity of the family life of these individuals becomes clearer upon examining the multitude of ways they share their economic resources. The majority has multiple sources of income. This does not mean that they have extra amounts of money. On the contrary, in most cases it means they have to have several jobs in order to keep an acceptable standard of living. Simultaneously, they work toward maintaining their family relations, which have value for financial and emotional support. A man who has been working for the government and now is retired and receives a pension, for instance, might have additional financial help from his grown children who live either with him or keep in close touch. A woman, for instance, who might be called a housewife can simultaneously be called "self-employed." She and her two unmarried daughters raise various kinds of poultry in their house. The production of their joint economic activities is sold in the market or consumed by them to replace what could have otherwise been bought from the market. At the same time the family receives the pension of their deceased father. The daughters give their support too when they are employed outside home for various periods. Another example is a woman who is employed by the government and simultaneously receives a pension for her deceased husband. In this chapter I will identify each person by his or her main source of income, that is, that source which constitutes the largest part of financial support for the person concerned. But it is important to keep in mind that this source is rarely adequate to support an individual separated from the family.

All the persons interviewed work to keep their family relationships alive. They exchange gifts and loans, for instance in their constant visitations and frequent meetings. Further, the relationships between parents and adult children remain vital for the support of either side. For example, two men in their mid-forties are still unmarried and stay at their parents' house. An adult female can stay even longer when unmarried at that age. Married children, especially women, would go back to their parents' homes if they were divorced or widowed. They would do this if they cannot live independently because of financial or other social conditions. Women, for instance, can be criticized if they live alone even if they can afford to do so. The vast majority of the individuals included (30, or 75 percent) are married and live with their children. Three adult males whose ages are thirty, forty-two, and forty-five are living with their parents. Being married and having children is predominantly the social event associated with leaving the parents' home in order to stay in a separate house. A woman whose husband works abroad and is unable to support her had to stay with her mother and two unmarried sisters. The husband's parents did not support the wife and expected her to leave her marital home to return to her own family.

No wonder then if the family (*al-'ā'ilah*), which means people connected by kin relations and living together and sharing their economic resources, is central in the lives of all the persons interviewed. There is a peculiar meaning of the concept of *al-'ā'ilah* in Arabic. First, it is derived from the Arabic root *'awala*, which means "to support." Other meanings refer to particular voices uttered in times of pain. As such, the term *al-'ā'ilah* suggests meanings of intimacy and simultaneously implies a sense of concern and obligation to support the other members of the social unit (al-Zabidi 1965). As I described in the previous chapters, *al-'ā'ilah* is associated with a strong sense of obligation and expectation which lasts after marriage. *Al-'ā'ilah* is based on physical and emotional connections by means of which individuals identify themselves and recognize the others and thus it is directly connected to the definitions of the body-self in health and illness.

All people in this survey consider themselves as having been ill with *'iḍḍaghṭ* for a period between two to twenty years. All the individuals received their diagnoses from medical specialists. Thirty of them suffered from other physical pains for a variety of periods. But only five of those connect their illnesses of *'iḍḍaghṭ* primarily to their other physical problems. Everyone, however, referred to emotional factors as the underlying causes of their illnesses including *'iḍḍaghṭ*. The reference to the physiological reasoning was understood in purely technical terms quoted from the patients' conversations with doctors.

Very few of the individuals explicitly question the validity of the term *'iḍḍaghṭ* as a label for their illness. For coping with this illness, however, all of them mobilize a variety of interpretations, therapeutic measures, and other methods and strategies which emphasize the plural character of the medical system. My argument is that all these complex therapies, which include religious, biochemical, or herbal remedies, constitute the discourse on *'iḍḍaghṭ*.

The idea of "social free association" used by Good (1977: 39) is particularly helpful here in depicting the various clusters of social experiences associated with *'iḍḍaghṭ*. Good's work is premised on the idea that "medical language, whatever its source, acquires meaning specific to a particular social and cultural context and in turn integrates illness and cure deeply into that context" (Good 1977: 31). The meaning of an illness term is "generated socially as it is used by individuals to articulate their experiences of conflict and stress, thus becoming linked to typical syndromes of stresses in the society." (Good 1977: 39). As such, Good tries to identify whether there is a distinctly Iranian network of meaning around the problem of heart distress. In this context, he inquires why seemingly heterogeneous anxieties such as contraception, pregnancy, old age, interpersonal problems, money worries are all associated with one illness. To explore such a framework Good's method involves listing the factors mentioned as causing a particular illness, then focusing on the meaning of the terms that describe those causes to identify the semantic links that bring them together. A diagram is drawn to illustrate these links. The ultimate aim of this method is to reveal the "semantic fields" associated with "clusters of experiences" linked to more basic structural elements of the society.

Furthermore, Good illustrates that the terms are ultimately linked to social symbols of power that crosscut heterogeneous fields and phenomena. Good uses several theoretical works concerned with symbolic analysis, the most important of which is Turner (1967) who treats ritual symbols as "forces" in social interaction. Ritual symbols represent social experiences and reveal the ideological or normative principles most fundamental to the society. In this way the terms used to describe illness experience include and link physical sensations of abnormality in the heart and feelings of anxiety, sadness, and anger, to larger issues occurring in the social environment such as female sexuality and oppression in daily life.

Turner describes the properties, or rather the functions, of the ritual symbols as those of *condensation*, *unification of disparate significata*, and *polarization of meaning*. Condensation refers to the process where a single symbolic formation represents diverse things and actions. The meanings of these elements are interlinked to appear as one unit because they possess equivalent qualities. Finally, and most importantly, each symbol has two distinct poles of meaning. The first refers to collective elements including the principles of social organization and the norms and values inherent in structural relationships. The other pole has natural or physiological phenomena or processes. In summary, Turner calls the first pole "ideological," and the second "sensory." The ideological pole is concerned with guidance and control via the use of shared norms and values. It represents the associational, domestic, and political unity and continuity of the social group. The sensory pole is concerned with the desires, feelings, and emotions and closely connected to frank, even flagrant physiological entities such as blood, semen, urine, etcetera (Turner 1967: 28–29, emphasis original).

My research is similar to Good's work in Iran. Zaina's illness, for example, brings her physical sensations (shaking like a waterskin) together with her perceptions of her position in the family and her precarious economic conditions. Zaina was not sure that *'iḍḍaghṭ* truly represents her suffering. Others, however, attempt to use the socially recognized category of unwellness so to speak. They reformulate its explanation and then link it to their most immediate concerns. I argue that the patients suffering from *'iḍḍaghṭ* in Cairo creatively *remake this term to accommodate their most pressing emotions of 'izza'al rooted in their perceived oppressive daily life. As a result, a network of meanings that refer to social experiences associated with 'iḍḍaghṭ is constituted.* As Good, I argue that this image has the power to help patients to evaluate their living conditions and thus their health status and life as a whole.

Causes for *'iḍḍaghṭ* were described by a total of forty-eight terms that were repeated 144 times throughout my different conversations with all the patients. Table 3.3 summarizes these causes under ten central terms. Figure 3.1 depicts how these terms are linked. The term *al-za'al* (painful anger) accounts for the largest proportion of the causes mentioned. It is directly connected to problems of the family life, the material hardships the members undergo expressed by some as *dughut al-hayaah* (pressures of life), and understood by others as a result of social injustice. This cluster of terms (including Nos. 1, 2, 4, 5 and 7) make up 75 percent of the terms associated with *'iḍḍaghṭ*. The rest of the terms referring to notions of pollution, other diseases, and that *'iḍḍaghṭ* is God-given make up for the rest, as will be discussed below.

Social Pressures of *'izza'al*

Figure 3.2 depicts the semantic links between the different terms used in the first domain of causes. Using people's words, the figure is diagrammed into a set of clusters and arrows where the clusters are factors perceived as relevant

Table 3.3. Causes of ʻiḍḍaghṭ

No.	Causes of ʻiḍḍaghṭ	Times Used	%
1.	*ʻizzaʻal* and *Katm* (painful anger and suppression of feelings of sadness, concern, excessive thinking, disgust, frustration, irritation, tension, worry)	48	33.3%
2.	*Al-ʻiyaal* (family stress due to increasing demands and need for regulating roles of different members)	25	17.4%
3.	*Al-ʻaya* (other diseases including hereditary predisposition, diabetes, kidney problems, heart problems, various kinds of surgeries, and smoking)	20	13.9%
4.	*Al-faqr* (lack or insufficiency of material resources required to set a life as required by social class, including shortage or unavailability of living space)	18	12.5%
5.	*ḍūghūṭ ḥayāh* (social pressures due to increasing prices and ever high social expectations)	11	7.64%
6.	*Talawwuth* (pollution of food, air, and water, and the effect of the contraceptive pill)	7	4.86%
7.	*Al-zulm (*social injustice)	6	4.20%
8.	*Al-tawattur* (fatigue due to overwork including stress, tension due to competition)	5	3.40%
9.	*Lamsah* and *Hassad* (spirit possession and evil eye)	4	2.8%
Total		144	100%

for the aetiology, pathophysiology, and outcome, and the arrows represent the causal relationships perceived to engendering *'iḍḍaghṭ*.

Unemployment—Insecurity—Worry—Interpersonal Problems—Higher Sensitivity—Nervousness—*zaʻal*—*ʻiḍḍaghṭ*

This is the most common causative scheme of *'iḍḍaghṭ* in Cairo. Problems of marital and family tensions are linked to an inability to meet material demands due to insufficient income. The difficulties ensuing from these circumstances lead to the feelings of insecurity or fear, worry, frustration, discontent, disgust, etcetera. *'Izza'al* (anger) grows under these circumstances and feelings. People who mention *'izza'al* as the main cause of their illness feel they are generally more sensitive than others. They think their feelings of *'izza'al* are due to the fact that they are more sensitive both emotionally and morally: "I cannot see things done wrongly and remain indifferent, I get angry, others don't, I am just more sensitive than others," one patient explains. The element of pressure here is linked directly to the moral constitution of the persons involved. When coupled with the other cultural category of *al-katm*, a persistent condi-

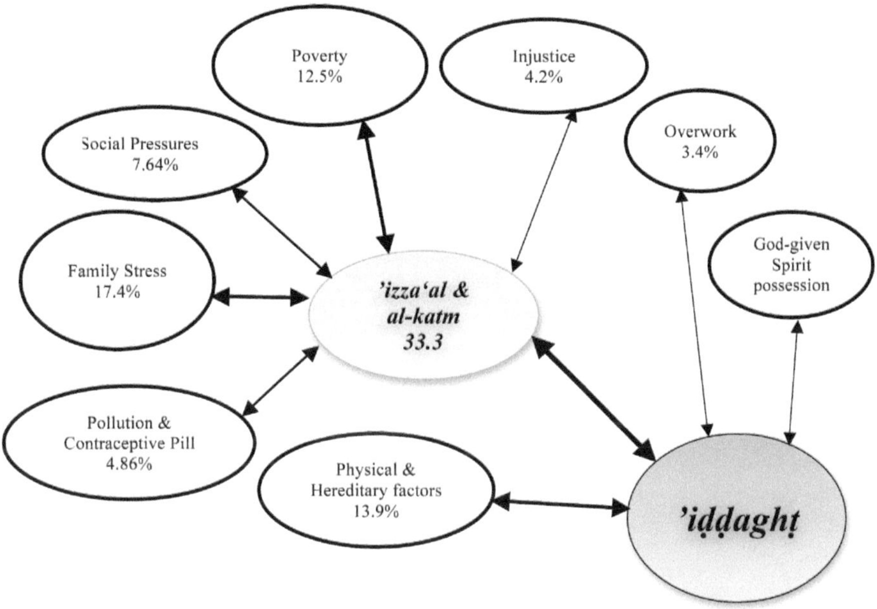

Figure 3.1. Causal Links of *'iḍḍaghṭ*

tion of *'izza'al* breeds sickness. *Al-katm* means blocking someone's breath (*nafas*), which represents preventing people from speaking out their feelings and frustrations. This element directly links to the notion of *al-nafs* with roots in the language and tradition of society as discussed earlier in this study. My argument is that *al-nafs* is the recipient of life conditions and thus represents the larger issue of "the oppression of the daily life." When a person falls ill with *'iḍḍaghṭ* in Cairo, people explain the onset of the disease by saying: "it got so hard on his *nafs* (*si'bit 'alaih nafsuh*)." In conclusion, the element of "oppressive daily life," also emphasised by Good (1977) is one ultimate pool of the causes underscored by all the interpretations of *'iḍḍaghṭ*.

The narratives above provide concrete examples for this interpretation. The material demands of Abu Hassan's family are perceived as being far beyond his ability to meet. Coupled with the persistent deterioration of the economic situation, these perceptions provided the reason for a continuous state of tension and led to a host of feelings of discontent. Although he did not show signs of *'izza'al*, evidence of factors engendering this feeling in his family was abundant.

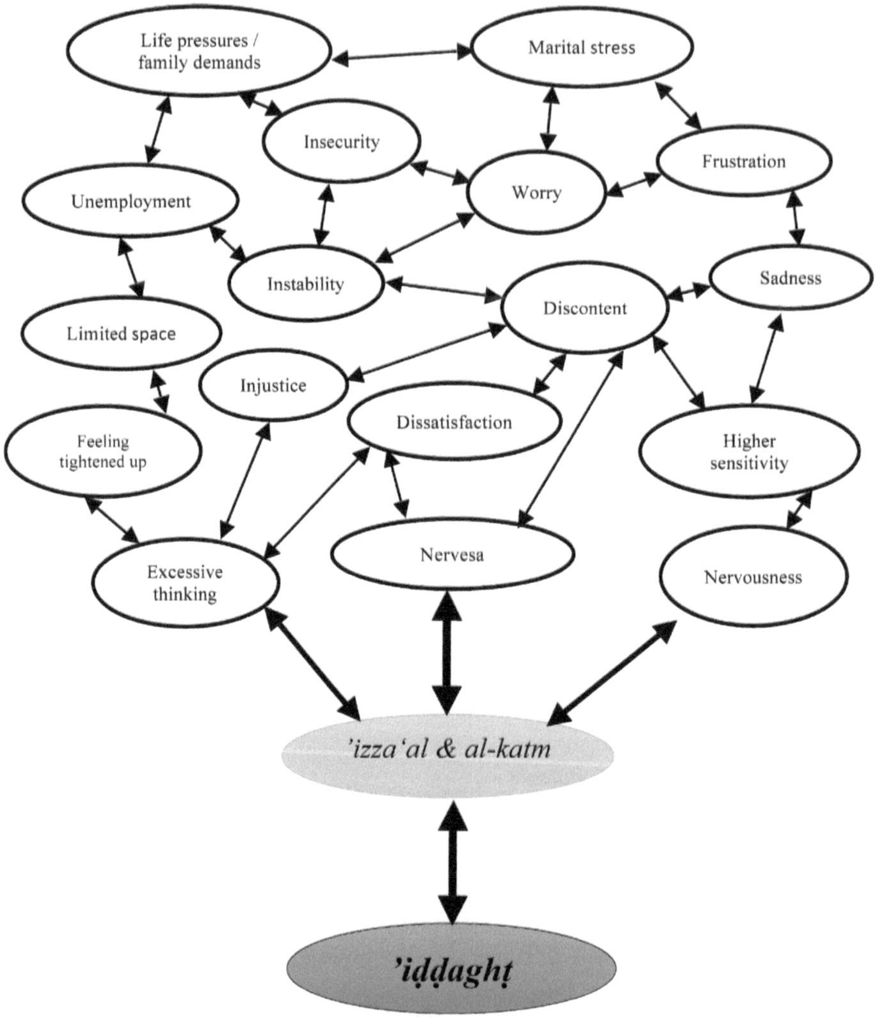

Figure 3.2. Social Pressures as Linked *'iḍḍaghṭ*

His being the head of the household and husband gives him enough grounds to withdraw into himself and thus control the impact of the adverse conditions. This privilege is not available to his wife who continues to bear the responsibility of managing the whole household, which represents the pressure of her life.

Pressures of Life—Injustice—Excessive Thinking—Discontent—Nerves—*za'al—katm—'iḍḍaghṭ*

These linked causes apply mostly to people such as Dr. Fawzi and Madame Farida. The "pressures" they mean are more for keeping up with their middle-class expectations than striving to make ends meet as in the case of Abu and Um Hassan. The elements of *'izza'al* in their case are slightly different from those of Abu and Um Hassan. That Dr. Fawzi was not treated fairly in his workplace connects to meanings of social inequality and his inability to challenge those. His wife's feelings of fury (*hamaq*) and the fact that she suffered from *katm* (blocking her own breath) bring her into contrast with Um Hassan, who is very outspoken about her reasons for discontent with everyday life. Madame Farida said she felt relieved when she screamed her anger out.

If we treat *'iḍḍaghṭ* as a symbol representing the above three processes outlined by Turner (1967), I would argue with Turner that in the context of my research, this social condition is perceived a "compromise formation" between the collective needs for social control on the one hand, and individual drives that threaten, if they are carried too far, to result in a breakdown of that control on the other (Turner 1967: 35–38). The compromise is implied by the meanings of the complex feelings of *'izza'al*.

Limited Space—Feeling Tightened Up—Dissatisfaction—Nerves— za'al—katm—'iḍḍaghṭ

This is one of the most common explanations of *'iḍḍaghṭ* in Cairo. The case of Abu and Um Hassan is a good example for a relatively large number of people living in a space perceived as too small. Furthermore, the issue of limited space goes far beyond people's homes. The city, its streets, buses, offices, apartments, and schools are perceived as being overcrowded and people in many contexts refer to the suffocating density of human activities. The case of Dr. Fawzi is a good example for this link where his complaints are not strictly about the space of his house but the city as a whole. *Zaḥma* (crowded) is a household term similar to *'iḍḍaghṭ*; the two are often mentioned together. I often heard references being made to Cairo's streets as suffocating (*mackhnū'ah*). Once I told a taxi driver that I was doing research on *'iḍḍaghṭ*. He immediately said while pointing to the congested streets: "*aṣli ḍaghṭ al-balad 'awi*" (because the city's pressure is too high), "how," he continued, "could you then expect us not to have *'iḍḍaghṭ*, such things set one's blood on fire" (*bitiḥra'iddam*). Clearly, crowdedness and spatial pressure are set in direct connection with individuals' own bodies and sense of health. This issue brings into focus the link between the body and environment and how the feelings about both are intrinsically interwoven. The notion of *dī'ah* (tightness), for example, is used in various contexts such as going though an economic hardship or living in a space that is inadequately small, or going through narrow and crowded streets. We notice here how the medical language of tightened blood vessels is extended to express problems in social life.

God-Given—*'iḍḍaghṭ*

This link has been mentioned by a very small number of people. It has always been mentioned in a list of other causes of social pressures and *'izza'al*. The explanation of *'iḍḍaghṭ* in Cairo is dominated by the search for ways to express social problems perceived as having adverse effects on health. When belief in misfortune is mentioned it points to the person's share in life that is laden with a higher possibility of falling sick due to factors of poverty and underprivilege.

Pollution and *'izza'al*

Figure 3.3 depicts the semantic links between the notion of *'iḍḍaghṭ* and pollution including environmental pollution and the effects of the contraceptive pill.

In the last few decades Cairo has witnessed a great amount of industrialization and population growth. Many factories were built in and around the city after the start of the open-door economic policy in the mid-1970s. Simultaneously, the city's population increased many fold. In addition to the already high birth rate in the city there has been a steady flow of rural immigrants who look for better jobs and places to live. These developments have placed an immense

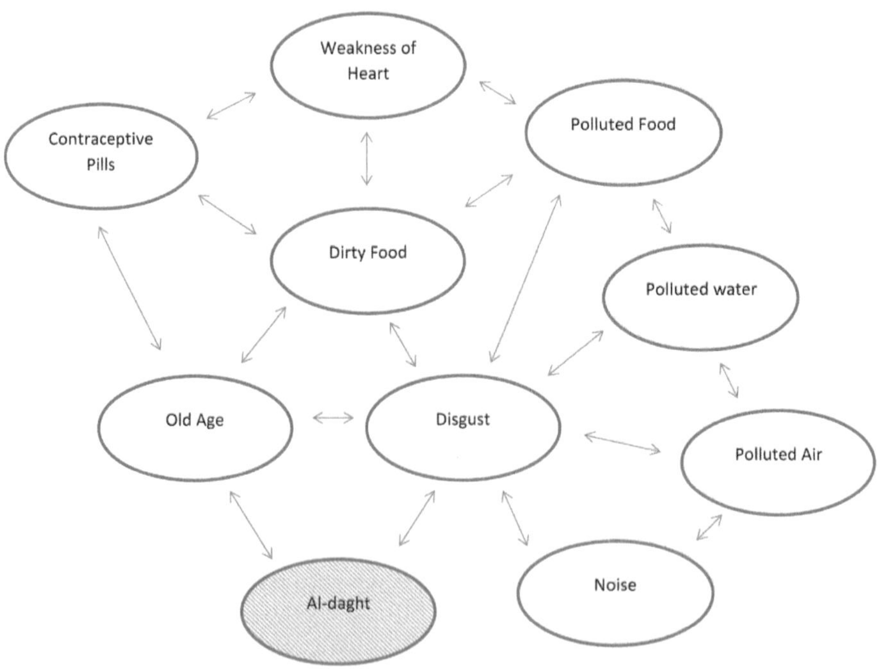

Figure 3.3. Pollution linked *'iḍḍaghṭ*

amount of pressure on the city's various facilities including the water system and transportation. The number of cars in the city increased manyfold, which further exacerbated the problem of air pollution and noise. In the morning one can literally see clouds of grey air around the Nile due to the humidity and increased air pollution. It is no coincidence then that many of my respondents replied to my question about the relevance of pollution to *'iḍḍaghṭ* by saying that the general condition of the city "burns their blood" or "place their nerves on fire." Both physicians and laypersons have quoted pollution as a cause *'iḍḍaghṭ*. The medical discourse is preoccupied with identifying the kind of chemicals spread in the air and water. Meanwhile, the general public, including the patients included in this study, emphazises its feeling of disgust and unrest as problems underlying its physical sensation of fatigue or exhaustion, which is also linked to old age. Both are causes of *'iḍḍaghṭ* and are linked to the notion of decay.

Pollution—Disgust—Fatigue—Old age—'iḍḍaghṭ*—The Contraceptive Pill—Weakness of the Heart—Sadness—*'iḍḍaghṭ

Exclusively women such as Zaina and Madame Farida mentioned this element. The general problem of pollution is connected to the belief that bad blood is retained due to the use of the contraceptive pill, which was originally intended to prevent pregnancy. Zaina's idea that her condition might have developed because she stopped giving birth is intrinsically connected to her general feeling of sadness about her oppressive daily life, generally characterised by insufficient material resources. In contrast, Madame Farida, who belongs to an educated middle class, connects similar feelings to her fury about her life circumstances in general.

'IḌḌAGHṬ: WHEN RATIONAL MEN FALL ILL

In Cairo two other terms are also used to express *'iḍḍaghṭ*. These are "*irtifā' ḍaghṭ al-dam*," (high blood pressure) and "hypertension." The medical practitioners mostly use this term. They rely on the clinical reading of the sphygmomanometers to decide whether somebody is ill or not. All practitioners, however, report that hypertension is difficult to explain and many cases are ultimately inconclusive. It thus remains subject of debate and experimental therapies. The physicians refer to inexplicable cases by the label "essential hypertension." They constantly mentioned the term in English. This is when the condition of abnormal blood pressure cannot be ascribed to one or a set of specific physical malfunctions. In treating hypertension, physicians keep experimenting with different therapies until one works. A prominent physician used the analogy of dressmaking to describe this process of experimentation. He said: "physicians in hypertension are like tailors, they sew up specific treatments for specific individuals." He meant that physicians always combine different kinds of therapeutic measures in their prescriptions. Each specific combination is good for a specific group of individuals characterized by specific constellations of symptoms. The processes of prescribing therapies are highly speculative according to this physician. Meanwhile, the patients' interpretations and therapies are not always limited to those of the physicians. The two kinds of explanations however overlap in important ways. The physicians who suffer from *'iḍḍaghṭ* are also engaged in processes of extensive social and moral evaluations. In result, no abstract and total explanation of *'iḍḍaghṭ* can be found in any single case. The syndrome is a product of a social discourse whose concepts are used in a variety of contexts.

In theory however, the physicians in Cairo ascribe high blood pressure to various physical factors such as ageing, obesity, heart disease, kidney problems, etcetera, or to long-term psychological stress. Very few, if any, show interest in identifying how these problems are perceived in cultural terms. This lack of interest is related to the long reliance of the Egyptian medical establishment on biomedical definitions. Biomedicine is the most powerful therapeutic system with an unrivaled amount of authority. It is the system which was entrusted early on by the national elite who subsequently discredited, at least officially, their long-standing inherited plural medical system (see Gran 1979).

A few years ago a number of academics and practitioners set up a nationwide nongovernmental organization called The Egyptian Society for Hypertension. The society's goal is "to reduce the incidence rates of hypertension and its complications as well as the mortality and disability resulting from high blood pressure among Egyptians" (The Egyptian Society for Hypertension 1997: 1). Shortly after it started the society conducted a survey, in 1995, to estimate the prevalence of hypertension in Egypt. The survey assumes that normal blood pressure is around "systolic pressure ≥ 120 mmHg and/or diastolic pressure ≥ 90 mmHg, and/or reported treatment with one or more anti-hypertensive medications" (Ibrahim et al. 1995). It uses the concept of hypertension and never mentions any other culturally based term. The survey is also a good example of the assumption that biomedical research should produce cross-culturally valid results. The survey was designed and conducted in collaboration with an American team and set out to further analyze sets of variables in their relationship to the occurrence of hypertension. The variables include bilharzia and "skin colour" (Ashour et al. 1995: 884). The study recognizes the relevance of variables such as education and income as parameters for social status. But it fails to grasp the circumstances of the majority of Egyptians. For example, it proposes to further look at "relevant variables unique to the Egyptian population (e.g., presence of electricity and air-conditioning)" (*ibid.*). Air-conditioning, it needs to be mentioned, is an irrelevant factor in most Egyptians' lives, but does play a more prominent role in the upper middle classes' imagination especially in their assumptions about stress (see Young 1980). Air-conditioning might have been considered a sign of social class. The survey, however, does not make this relationship explicit. It is primarily concerned with purely clinical definitions of the disease.

'Iḍḍaghṭ has long been a theme in the press with a variety of comments from physicians and editors. The authority of medical science is always invoked by either quoting physicians or the medical studies and surveys they conduct. The media, however, have always to relate to experiences lived by the audience. *Al-Ahram*, the main and half-official newspaper, has *'iḍḍaghṭ* on its front page. It quotes the survey mentioned above to report that "31 percent of the Cairo population show the clinical signs of abnormally high blood pressure." The disease is presented as independent of individual consciousness and social position: "not all of those found with abnormal blood pressure are aware that they are ill," the paper warns. The principal researcher who led the team that conducted the survey, a prominent Cairo University cardiologist, is quoted:

> The causes of the prevalence of the disease are environmental factors such as noise (*ḍawḍā'*), lead pollution, smoking, overcrowding (*zuḥām*) and the morality of overcrowding (*'akhlāq al-zuḥām*) which lead to compression, besides other biological factors such as diabetes, obesity, and damage resulting from excessive table salt.

So physicians too joined in reproducing the popular model of *'iḍḍaghṭ* and in ways that sustain it as a morally laden space and an opportunity to express discontent. Many other ideas are published in the press. My argument is that physicians too use the traditional resources that enable people to speak about *'iḍḍaghṭ* as something representing the adverse life conditions of their selves, the families, communities, and society at large. *'Iḍḍaghṭ* in conclusion therefore is not a disease by itself. It gives people a chance to speak about how life is made dis-eased as it were. When physical causes are quoted to explain the incidence of high blood pressure for example like constricting blood vessels (*Al-Ahram* 19.10.1997), use of contraceptive pills (*Al-Wafd* 9.9.1996), and the genetic determination of the disease, they are placed in contexts of life conditions that are generally in decline. Pollution of both air and water too is suspected to increase the concentration of harmful chemicals in the blood (*Al-Ahram* 13.2.1997). No one though has demonstrated such relationship.

The causes cited in the press therefore are not totally different from those narrated by laypersons. Rather, both should be viewed as parts of a continuum that includes a professionalized language of disease at one end and a quasi-scientific language of unwellness at the other. The literate culture of Egypt has long provided many channels to link the text to the body, as I discuss in the introduction of this study. Means such as the mosque, the TV and radio, in addition to printed materials such as the self-help guide to be discussed next, are responsible for translating abstract professional concepts into cultural expressions accessible to many people. This process of translation brings medical concepts into close contact with inherited cultural concepts, a process of interaction responsible for developing, although not necessarily determining, the whole content of the popular culture.

Some of the commentaries diverge from the above explanatory schemes. *Al-Ahram* publishes a report that excessive anger (*al-ghaḍab*) and strain (*al-ham*) are the main causes of many heart diseases including *'iḍḍaghṭ* (*Al-Ahram* 24.12.1995). *Al-ghaḍab* is the formal Arabic synonym for a term used widely in the colloquial Egyptian dialect called *'izza'al*, which I will discuss below. The paper however advises sufferers of *'iḍḍaghṭ* to consult their physicians as frequently as possible and to use all means available, including old and new ones, to control this condition. Despite the seeming similarity to the colloquial term, the paper then falls back into a medicalized understanding of *'iḍḍaghṭ* that implicitly eschews mentioning the factors underlying the spread of feelings of anger and discontent. This example however shows that both the professional and popular terms are closely connected linguistically.

Another example is a self-help guide written by a physician and published as a low-priced booklet sold in many bookshops and newspaper stalls. The guide consists of a hundred pages with the title "If You Suffer From High Blood Pressure: Your Natural Therapy From Herbs And Nutrition." It combines elements of biomedicine that are occasionally introduced in close connection with religious concepts, moral advice, as well as herbal therapy. The author of the guide is a physician, Ayman al-Hussaini, who is introduced in the first pages as a graduate of the Islamic University of al-Azhar. The guide is an example that roughly exemplifies the composite therapeutic forms used for diagnosing and treating *'iḍḍaghṭ* in various sectors of society.

The cover of the guide consists of diagrams of the human circulatory system, a large picture of the heart drawn separately at the other corner of the cover. At the center of the heart is a small photograph showing how the instrument for measuring blood pressure fits onto an arm for testing. In the middle between the heart and the circulatory system emerges a rectangular shape surrounding a collection of assorted herbs. This cover represents a widely used pragmatic approach of interpretation and treatment of *'iḍḍaghṭ* by elements from different traditions.

The booklet contains ideas that are based on biomedical diagnosis and therapeutic methods originating in what the author calls "natural therapy" (*al-'ilāg al-tabī'i*). Along similar lines the booklet is organized in two parts. The first part defines blood pressure as a result of nervous, hormonal, or other physical causes such as kidney and heart problems. First, it suggests that people who are susceptible to *'iḍḍaghṭ* are those individuals whose parents have had the disease. The disease is hereditary (*wirāthi*). This explanation is now very common in biomedicine. Multimillion projects of research are put in service of gathering information on the genetic determination of various diseases. It is worth mentioning here that this search is not for a physical element that determines human health. Genes are codified systems of data the knowledge of which does not necessarily help reduce the ambiguity of causation. Socially speaking though, it operates to focus on singular bodies as suspects for causing disease. It distracts the attention from the social and cultural dimensions of the complaint involved.

Following this explanation that places blame on past generations is another that places the blame on the patients because they are "tense and competitive individuals." Sufferers of *'iḍḍaghṭ* are sometimes "engaged in dogfights over mundane gains" (*al-mutawattirūn wal mutanāfisūn: al-mutakaalibūn-'ala 'umūr al-dunya*) (*ibid.*: 18). Under this heading the author explains that such individuals are susceptible to different forms of psychological reactions such as *tawattur* (tension), *nafāth al-ṣabr* (running out of patience), *talahhuf* (sighing—which means people who sigh while impatiently waiting for things to be finished quickly). Such factors lead to high blood pressure which is widespread among people who compete for success in life, such as businessmen or those who work very hard (*ibid.*: 18). Obesity, increased salt intake, smoking, contraceptive pills, increased intake of tea and coffee, age, and sex are all known medical variables for *'iḍḍaghṭ* and are listed and briefly explained. At the end of this part the author describes how blood pressure is measured and the different medical meanings of its different signs.

The second part of the book contains the physician's advice and recommended therapies. First is to buy a sphygmomanometer and to keep track of one's blood pressure. Second is to reduce one's weight in case the patient is overweight. Third is to do physical exercises. Fourth is to try to be vegetarian. Fifth is to avoid a high salt intake. Sixth is to eat food rich in potassium and calcium. Seventh is to avoid taking boiled tea or very hot tea and coffee. The eighth piece of advice is "Don't talk much," which is advice supported by research conducted at an American university, according to the author. The author reports that "researchers believe that the everyday talking of people is often connected to increased heart activity which might lead to an unexpected increase in blood pressure during these conversations." Ninth is "not to take medicines for *'iḍḍaghṭ* in a random way" but in the exact way the doctor recommends. The tenth and eleventh pieces of advice are suggestions for regular physical checkups. The twelfth suggestion urges the reader to "try to live happily as much as possible." The author quotes a study from a hospital in New York. The study found out that worries and tension have negative physical effects if they are experienced outside one's own home. Those effects however become less if the tension is experienced inside one's own home. The author takes this conclusion to advise patients of increased blood pressure to "try to live happily . . . and if [they] have to be tense then they should try to be so inside the home" (*ibid.*: 53). Finally, the author implies that high blood pressure can spread through long contact between people, such as between partners. Partners have similar blood pressure because they are exposed to similar amounts of tension. As a result, the therapeutic advice relies on heterogeneous methods and ideas impossible to classify under a single category, but within the particular experience and cultural background of the author.

Causes of *'iḍḍaghṭ* are sought in the individual body: the amount of salt in food, drinking tea and coffee, etcetera. Social relations are also implied by the situations that lead to tension, competition, and anger. The physician's advice considers simultaneously controlling both kinds of cause as essential for preventing *'iḍḍaghṭ*. For factors with physical effects he calls for certain kinds of diet that would involve changing the individual's eating habits. For factors that obviously emanate in social relations, he simply uses moral meanings that condemn certain behaviors such as competition. Human interaction represented by talking and engaging in conversation is construed as one factor leading to ill health.

The remaining sections of the second part are concerned with advice on the herb therapies that may contribute to controlling blood pressure. Throughout this section the physician mentions the biochemical and nutritional characteristics of the herbs which are always labeled with their Arabic as well as Latin names and explained by referring to studies written in Arabic as well as in English. In addition, the physician includes whatever support comes from the Quran or from common wisdom, or from Chinese or Ancient Egyptian medicine. In explaining the therapeutic effects of ginger, for example, he includes the Quranic verse: "And they will be given to drink there a cup [of wine] mixed with *ganzabīl* (ginger, etc.); a spring there called *salsabīl*" (The Quran, cited in al-Hussaini 1993: 65).

It is worth mentioning here that many patients mention terms very similar to the physician's. A closer look, however, reveals that the patients' terms are situated differently and thus have different meanings. Patients, for example, give the element of "talking" a whole different meaning and role. Many interviewees mention that their illness developed because they suppressed, or were made to suppress, their feelings and words. This practice of suppression is possible through the cultural category of *katm*, to be described in the narratives below. Furthermore, unlike the recommendation of the author, many see their homes and families as the place to contract the disease, rather than to realise recovery. There are several other differences in the narratives to follow. These case examples include physicians as well as laypersons complaining of *'iḍḍaghṭ*. They present different and new ideas inspired not only by abstract models, but also by practical experiences contributing to the formation of the local biologies.

Good (1977) argues that the meaning of medical language depends on the particular historical, sociocultural context in which that language is generated. (*ibid*: 31). Furthermore, he suggests that that language is "the medium through which vicious and life-threatening power struggles are engaged" (B. Good 1995: 14). So, what happens when particular terms such as *'iḍḍaghṭ* are linked to body sensations, feelings and social experiences specific to the lives of the individuals suffering from the illness? How do people arrive to the conclusion that *'iḍḍaghṭ* is their main problem? What terms are mentioned next to the term *'iḍḍaghṭ*? What are the meanings of these terms and what do they imply about the different pressure (*ḍūghūt*) of life experienced in Cairo?

THINKING ABOUT HIGH BLOOD PRESSURE AND SUFFERING FROM 'IḌḌAGHṬ

Some of the health practitioners who have abnormal readings of high blood pressure like to identify their illness with the clinical reality they construct and by which they live. The relation between their professional concepts of disease and the popular term of *'iḍḍaghṭ* remains unexplored. Dr. Sherif is a senior physician in his late fifties. He worked for the governments in both Egypt and Saudi Arabia for many years before he returned to work for the private sector. He says his blood pressure has been abnormally high for the last five years. He retired within the last three years. I met Dr. Sherif in his house in an upper-middle-class quarter of Cairo where he lives with his wife and two sons. I was introduced to them by one of their close relatives. In explaining the causes behind his illness Dr. Sherif said:

> I was the manager of a private hospital and there was great amount of work and many responsibilities involved in running the place. Hypertension is associated with extra effort and long hours of work. Stress associated with a career is the primary cause associated with high blood pressure.

In order to control his illness and physical discomfort Dr. Sherif takes medicines in a highly disciplined manner. He regulates his meals, which his wife cooks, and sleeps at predefined times. He says he keeps away from the details of everyday life and leaves these to his wife and children:

> I became less concerned with the details of everyday life and the pain of the head (*wag' aldimāgh*). Now, I read books most of the day. I go for walks. I don't get into arguments with other people. All this gives me great amount of mental comfort (*rāḥit al-bāl*).

Dr. Sherif's illness narrative is a good example for a reified medical explanation (Helman 1985) common in empiricist stress researches (Young 1980). Furthermore, this explanation is attached to privileges, such as resignation from social life, inaccessible to the majority of the population (see Frankenberg 1980). Other people who have high blood pressure think it is caused by their living under a variety of negative feelings such as excessive *za'al* (painful anger), *ghaḍab* (rage), *'aṣabiyya* (nervousness) intensive thinking (*tafkīr*) or *tawattur* (tension) as we will see below.

Other physicians keep shifting between their professional models and what can be called the "popular" model of *'iḍḍaghṭ*. High blood pressure simply cannot represent all the complex feelings and emotions lived by everybody, including the health practitioners. As Frank (1997) argues, with modernist biomedicine it has become not only possible, but also necessary, for ill people to tell their own stories (*ibid.*: 149). This necessity leads into the concept of *'iḍḍaghṭ*, which offers a space that combines the complex physical, emotional, and social aspects of life, as we will see in the following cases. Such physicians agree on the causes listed by Dr. Sherif. But their clinical reality is only part of a larger world that they share with their patients. Although few, the moral and social dimensions mentioned above are instructive about what is left unspoken in the physicians' clinical official discourse on high blood pressure. I argue that *'iḍḍaghṭ* speaks from that region of silence, including the cultural meanings relevant to people's everyday circumstances.

The physicians' practices reveal that they are not free of doubts and debates on the underlying causes and meanings of this condition. Dr. Khalil is a prominent physician and director of a major hospital in Cairo. I met Dr. Khalil many times while visiting his workplace in order to interview and follow up a number of individuals visiting or admitted to his hospital. Throughout my visits to the hospital I kept meeting Dr. Khalil in both casual and planned manners: in the gardens of the health unit, in the outpatient clinic, and, most frequently, in his office. The views I collected from Dr. Khalil and other physicians are crucial in illustrating the shifting grounds and the physicians' multiple voices about the aetiologies of *'iḍḍaghṭ*.

Dr. Khalil long promised to give me some time for an interview in which he would deliver his view on what *'iḍḍaghṭ* is "really" about. As a sign of support and sympathy he answered my demand to interview him:

> That will help you to say the right things in your university examinations. Hypertension is just a very well-known illness and we know not only what happened to the patients but also what will happen to them.

In the interview he stated what many other physicians and health professionals in Cairo once said. What was interesting, however, were Dr. Khalil's views about hypertension that I collected during my casual meetings with him. In the garden of the hospital, for example, he argued: "Hypertensives, akh! The *real* problems of these people are not food and salt, they are the suffocating conditions of life under which people have to live." This view is a crucial part of the individuals' and families' explanatory methods for *'iḍḍaghṭ* and obviously goes far beyond the boundaries of conventional medical explanation and thus into the territory of the society in which Dr. Khalil and other physicians live. The views of the physicians are complex, representing their training at medical school and work experiences encompassed in their cultural backgrounds.

Dr. Khalil's thoughts became clearer through the words of his co-worker, Dr. Bassam, who is ill with high blood pressure. He is in his late forties and his blood pressure has been "badly elevated in the last ten years," as he puts it. I met Dr. Bassam several times when he was stopping by Dr. Khalil's office to communicate with him about various matters of work, or to drink tea. Dr. Khalil kept jokingly suggesting that I should take Dr. Bassam as a "typical case" for my research project. He meant that Dr. Bassam is a case that has been properly diagnosed and controlled and which illustrates different aspects of the disease. Dr. Bassam first reiterated more or less the same explanation as Dr. Khalil for his illness. He confirmed that he had constricted blood vessels, which developed as a result of increased stress and long hours of work. But on another occasion both doctors agreed that the illness is also related to social conditions which Dr. Bassam has experienced, especially during his marital life. Dr. Bassam once explained:

> I married twice; both marriages were unsuccessful and ended with divorce. In both cases I was unable to meet the financial demands of my wives, it was difficult . . . you know, lots of pressures lead to madness not only to hypertension.

Dr. Bassam's attempts to explain his health problems illustrate how *'iḍḍaghṭ* is a field that involves several explanatory schemes next to the biomedical category of high blood pressure. If taken as a whole, Dr. Bassam's explanations clearly cross the boundaries of professional schemes he mentioned earlier, into what can be called "popular explanatory models" that include a complex of emotional, spiritual, and physical elements, all related to Dr. Bassam's life, including his financial and social problems.

But what does enable Dr. Bassam to meaningfully link different dimensions of *'iḍḍaghṭ*? Is there a distinctively Egyptian framework to interpret this syndrome and which transcends biomedicine? What other terms do people use to reflect on their illness? Throughout my research, I was intrigued by one term commonly used to describe "the mood" or "the temperament" of people called *'il-mizāg*. If a person's *mizāg* is "*ma'dūl*" or balanced, that person must be feeling very well and have *rāḥit al-bāl*, or the peace of mind to work, not only efficiently but also joyfully. The relevance of this term became evident as many of my interviewees explained *'iḍḍaghṭ* by the lack of harmony in their lives. As a therapy, many suggested providing them with social settings where they can feel some peace of mind, which is directly linked to meanings of *'il-mizāg*. The concept, according to a contemporary lexicon of Arabic used in Egyptian schools, originates in Greek-Islamic medicines where *il-mizāg* means the mixture of the four humors, that is, blood, black bile, yellow bile, and phlegm (*Magm' illughah al-'arabiyya*). A good balance between these four fluids means good health. Disturbing that balance results in disordered health. The meaning of this concept, of course, must have changed since the time when the texts on Islamic medicine were widely used. But its persistence in language points to its relevance for contemporary perceptions of health and illness.

In his review of original sources on Greek and Islamic medicines, Byron Good (1995) finds that blood and phlegm are the two most important humors in explaining diseases (*ibid.*: 88–115). In Egypt today we encounter blood being used as a metaphor to describe reactions to demanding situations, that is, those situations that require an ability to respond to various stimuli, related to events significant to the persons involved. *fār al-dam bidmāgi* (blood rushed up to my brain), for instance, is used to say "I was very angry as a result of a bad event, action, accident etcetera." To have such an unusual reaction indicates that the persons involved have a sense of honor causing them to act properly in situations where their integrity or upright morals are concerned or challenged. In contrast, the expression *ma'andūsh dam* (he is void of blood) is used to describe the inability to respond to provocative situations such as insults, especially those related to one's honor and pride.

In thought then, different qualities of blood are metaphorically used to express different states of being, including health and illness. Structurally speaking, the concept of tranquility or calm mind (*rāḥit bāl*) involves the favored conditions necessary for living in peace and thus in good health. In contrast concepts such as *'ala'* (distress) and *waga' dimāgh* (pain in the head) refer to unfavorable, although inevitable, circumstances leading to stirred blood (*fār al-dam bi-dmāghi*), and imply devalued conditions that lead to bad health and possibly illness.

But when do people decide they are ill with *'iḍḍaghṭ*? How is *'iḍḍaghṭ* interpreted? Are the causes sought inside or outside the body? Is the divide between the inside body and the outside relevant here? The statement "I have the pressure (*'andi 'iḍḍaghṭ*)" in Cairo refers to an already defined pressure as we will see below in the case examples. People rarely mention the clinical signs of high blood pressure when they speak about *'iḍḍaghṭ*. Many say they have *'iḍḍaghṭ* although they have never been tested for it. These statements invite ideas and feelings about the social and economic circumstances they live including their family life, their suppressed feelings of anger and dissatisfaction, the problems of their city, whose air and water are perceived as polluted and too crowded. All these settings are conceived of as existing in a state of imbalance reflected on people's sense of health. In this sense, the widely used expression: "I have the pressure" (*'andi 'iḍḍaghṭ*) points to complex social problems that happen to be conceived as pressures experienced in close connection to what happens inside the body.

POPULAR NOTIONS OF 'IḌḌAGHṬ

Sickness Narratives

The instances that link *'iḍḍaghṭ* to various social problems in Cairo are many. The following examples include many links through cultural terms and symbols lived by people coming from various social backgrounds.

Narrative No. 1

Dr. Fawzi and Madame Farida (she likes to be called Madame for its taste of middle-class cultural etiquette) are a couple in their mid-sixties and have been married for more than forty years. They place their experiences in close connection to the unbearable "pressures of life" connected to their unrealized middle-class aspirations. Most prominent in their experiences are Dr. Fawzi's career aspirations, unattained due to unfair treatment at work, and Madame Farida's sense of stress, tension, and worry resulting from her responsibilities as wife and mother. The couple's experiences, however, are interconnected and should be viewed in the context of their common life circumstances.

The couple live in a neighborhood on the fringes of Cairo that once was a fashionable winter and health vacation spot but has long since lost its former glory, and even its middle-class aspirations of the more recent past. Over the past few decades the neighborhood has become home to a number of severely polluting industrial enterprises, including cement and asbestos manufacturing. In comparison to the majority of Cairene families, Dr. Fawzi's family is relatively well off. Dr. Fawzi, his wife, and eighteen-year-old daughter live in a rented apartment. He has a doctorate in geology, which he obtained in the 1960s in the United States. The social prestige attached to such a degree is considerable. Upon his return to Egypt he joined the government service and was eventually promoted to a high position in the Egyptian bureaucracy. Some years ago he retired from his public post but continues working as a part-time consultant for a ministry. Within his reach and setting, Dr. Fawzi is not completely satisfied with his material conditions. He feels he could have done better in terms of his bureaucratic career. He states with certain bitterness: "the ladder up was too high, I was at some point simply pushed out." Madame Farida has a high school diploma, which is rather unusual in Cairo for women of her age and clearly indicates the family's deep middle-class roots. She has never worked outside the house. Her main job in life, as she explains, was to take care of her children and house. The couple have six children, all of whom, except for the youngest daughter, are married and have left their parents' home. All of the five married children have university degrees. Dr. Fawzi, his wife, and daughter live off his pension and earnings as a consultant. They do not receive support from the married children. Dr. Fawzi remarked semi-ironically on his married children: "I just hope they will not ask me for help."

Both Dr. Fawzi and Madame Farida are currently taking medication for a variety of illnesses including *'iḍḍaghṭ*. Dr. Fawzi was first diagnosed with *'iḍḍaghṭ* some two decades ago when in his late forties. Ever since then he has been on medication. There were no special events or conditions relating to the onset of his illness. He merely recounts the day when he was walking down a street and all of a sudden felt the sensation of a strong headache and general weakness. He immediately consulted one of his doctor friends whose clinic was nearby at the time of the incident. The most serious "brush" with illness in Dr. Fawzi's life was, however, clearly related to a special event: his heart disease, which started with angina and was followed by a heart attack, took place shortly after he had been denied promotion. He had at the time believed that he deserved this promotion and that it was his turn in line to receive it. Shortly after this incidence of disease he also developed Bell's palsy, which Dr. Fawzi refers to as partial paralysis (*shalal niṣfi*). Dr. Fawzi and his family and friends identify his diseases as a direct result of this denial of the expected promotion.

Like many others in Cairo, Dr. Fawzi believes that disease in general and *'iḍḍaghṭ* in particular are the results of *dūghūṭ ḥayāh* (pressures of life). He identifies "economic pressure" as first and foremost among these. This type of pressure, of course, works as part of a vicious circle, as Dr. Fawzi notes, even the constantly rising prices of medication feed into the pressure that makes one sick. He further elaborates, "but it is all the demands of social life combined which made me sick." For him this is the particular result of his class position whereby he has to maintain class-based expectations with a budget that in reality no longer allows for that. Dr. Fawzi puts this pressure to reach for what is no longer possible for his family in relation to his present physical condition. He uses the term *'infi'āl* (best translated as "agitation or provocation associated with irritation") and *tawattur* (tension) to describe his sense of being out of control of his social and economic conditions, which he sees as being at the root of his physical suffering. His idea of how to deal with *'infi'āl* is through *īmān* (faith) and *qanā'ah* (content). He further explained that it is faith that enables him to live peacefully with disease and other hardships. Dr. Fawzi observes his prayers and a small dark spot on his forehead bears witness to this.

When I remarked, in more general terms, that I often wondered how people in Cairo really managed to cope with all sorts of hardships, he offered his explanation: "it is simply *baraka* and *satr* and these two can never come except from God and our belief in Him." *Baraka* is an immensely rich term covering the wider field of meaning related to blessing, and it also implies a very important notion of sharing. This notion holds that the goods of life can be increased if they are not strictly calculated; meaning that to give will engender blessing in itself and more so blessings of favors and goods returned. The notion of *baraka* further evokes the belief that all resources in the last instance come from God and hence carry an obligation for sharing. *Baraka* hence can come with sharing limited resources. For instance when small quantities of food are enough for many people it is believed that those foods have *baraka* in them. Similarly, *satr* (literally: covering) is the practice of negating one's own needs, to "cover" them so to speak, and also the practice of helping others in a hidden manner, that is, without showing off one's generosity.

In addition to biomedical treatments and his strong religious beliefs Dr. Fawzi also relies on herbal treatments recommended to him by friends. He regularly drinks *karkadieh* (a tisane made from dried hibiscus flowers) which is widely used for its effect in reducing blood pressure. As he has also been diabetic for a long time, he starts his day by eating a mixture of fenugreek, coriander, and lupine, mixed with honey. He eats this mixture and drinks *karkadieh* along with the pills which the doctor prescribed for him. Dr. Fawzi is very disciplined about the routine of taking his medication and keeping to his prescribed diet. Both he and his wife follow the doctor's advice, which is reinforced by their son, who is a general practitioner, with regard to the amount of fat, salt, sugar, and other spices they should consume. As much as Dr. Fawzi defends these dietary rules, there remains a grain of doubt about them in his mind: "these pills are only preventive of further damage, they can never cure what has already changed in the body." Dr. Fawzi's doctor son keeps up with his parents' health. When the need arises he refers him to various specialists who were his teachers at the medical school. Unlike the majority of Cairenes, Dr. Fawzi and his wife thus have access to some of the best of Cairo's facilities and practitioners. On the whole they have pieced together for themselves a unique and comprehensive system of treatments: faith, dietary rules, and the assistance of practitioners, and have found a way to live and cope with their health problems.

Madame Farida's initial encounter with *'iḍḍaghṭ* differs from her husband's in that it was at the much younger age of thirty. She has been taking medication ever since. She gave birth to three children after the onset of *'iḍḍaghṭ*, which has added further stress to her health. Madame Farida's treatment and rules, in particular her dietary rules, are less strict than those of her husband. She acknowledges the significance of controlling her diet but she usually breaks these regulations by taking more salt and spices on her food than recommended by her son. Unlike the husband she believes that what counts in the case of *'iḍḍaghṭ* is to live in a quiet and relaxed environment. Madame Farida largely believes in the medicine she takes and their remedying effects. She highly values the pills she is prescribed as the most effective means to guarantee a "comfortable" life with her illness. While she takes a number of herbs she refuses to ascribe any considerable healing effect to them. Madame Farida is not essentially in conflict with her husband's ideas. Her explanation of *'iḍḍaghṭ* varies significantly from her husband's, although she connects it to her feelings about economic needs as well as the tension associated with raising her children and making them succeed in their studies and lives. Instead of *'izza'al* she says her feeling was "*ḥama'*." *Ḥama'* literally means madness, but in this context it means any kind of irrational feeling connected to anger. In either case, *ḥama'* places anger outside the circle of rational behavior. Dr. Fawzi here interfered in his wife's talk: "mothers are more emotional than fathers and that is why the problems of children affect them more." It was clear that Madame Farida was the most involved of the pair with the children's studies and other problems. She is keen to stress that she is still carrying on with her children: "we took good care of our children not only until they completed their studies. We also ensured that they have good college degrees, marriages and jobs." Madame Farida perceives these sources of tension with relation to her children and family as being directly connected to her poor health because she used to hide her feelings: "I had always learned to hide my feelings of unhappiness until I fell ill. Only after that, I started to 'scream' my discontent out which gave me relief."

On the whole, Dr. Fawzi and Madame Farida like to assert firmly that their ill health can never be ascribed to one single cause, nor could it be cured, or at least controlled, through one single method. Their method of living with their sicknesses becomes conceivable through the words of Dr. Fawzi. He says:

> My work, my wife and children, my everyday life problems, from the amount of salary I receive to the traffic jam I get caught up in when I drive to my work, all are full of situations which "set my nerves on fire" (*bitiḥra' 'aṣābi*).

This complex set of methods of diagnosis and treatment constitutes the meaning of *'iḍḍaghṭ* in the lives of the couple. Their reliance on these therapeutic methods balances out the pressures and other problems perceived to cause their pains although they never help to heal them.

Narrative No. 2

So far I have described the views of practitioners and patients who come from middle-income groups. These views, however, are not essentially different from those of members of low-income groups in *Būlāq*. I argue that all groups are subject to the same discourse on *'iḍḍaghṭ* although in different degrees and contexts. My first encounter with the sufferers from *'iḍḍaghṭ* was with Zaina, who is a woman in her late thirties and mother of five sons and the [I assume she is his only wife] wife of a wage laborer. I met Zaina in the outpatient clinic of the general hospital in *Būlāq* where she collects her medicines. Her words connect her illness to her feelings about her home, husband, and children. They bring together complex meanings of uncertainty about the circumstances of her life, commitment to her children, her reproductive life, in addition to explanatory factors such as her feelings of disappointment and sadness:

> worrying about my children is a real *waga' dimāgh* (pain for my brain). Others even envy me because I have such five losers [her sons] although none of them makes even a penny. My husband is another headache. He has no stable job. He works one day and sits for two. I don't know, perhaps all my pain is because I was taking the contraceptive pills for three years. I really don't know. I could have been healthier had I continued conceiving and giving birth. In place of that, I am just disappointed, upset and sad.

In contrast to Dr. Sherif's narrative, Zaina does not accept *'iḍḍaghṭ* as representing her "real" pains,

> They [the physicians] say my problem is *'iḍḍaghṭ*. This is nonsense. I feel the problem in my heart. I no longer can hold my back upright . . . because my heart cannot bear my life circumstances anymore. When *'iḍḍaghṭ* comes to me, my body, especially my chest, feels like shaking like a waterskin (*'irba*).

I met Zaina only once. For some reason she stopped coming to the clinic before I could ask her if I could meet her family at home. Her thoughts however remained relevant throughout my research. They sum up many feelings and perceptions of the patients I met in different stages, such as in my in-depth research with the family of Abu Hassan in chapter 1, which constitutes the next narrative.

Narrative No. 3

Abu Hassan and Um Hassan (seventy and sixty-one years old respectively) have been married for over forty-five years and have eight living grown-up sons and daughters; four other children died in early childhood. Their life circumstances are similar to those of Zaina and illustrate many aspects about *'iḍḍaghṭ* lived by many people in *Būlāq* and similar quarters of Cairo. Their narrative illustrates how they view *'iḍḍaghṭ* as a characteristic of their general life circumstances, including the physical problems of the city they inhabit, such as a shortage of space and pollution. Their family problems and tensions are perceived as resulting from a shortage of economic resources. Most importantly, their general life circumstances lead to a complex set of feelings summed up under the common expression of anger (*'izza'al*) central to most of the narratives included in this study.

Abu Hassan retired from his job as a bookbinder ten years ago and now lives on his pension. He has been ill for the last ten years. Beside *'iḍḍaghṭ*, he suffers from rheumatic arthritis, gout (*nuqrus*), and diabetes (*sokkar*). Around the time of his retirement he suffered from the first symptoms of *'iḍḍaghṭ*. He remembers that at the time the family went through a severe economic crisis. He fell ill immediately after a major family fight, although he does not perceive this as the only cause of the disease. Abu Hassan's understanding of his illness illustrates the larger framework within which he understands his physical health. Multiple frustrations and disappointments in life, economic instability, combined with heightened irritation resulting from spatial pressure (*dī'ah*), bad or polluted food (*akl al-kimāwiyyāt*), noise (*dawsha*), pollution (*talawwus*) of the city, are factors, as Abu Hassan frequently points out, that cause people to fall sick. Such conditions and the feelings and impressions they engender can irritate the soul (*nafs*). All this is subsumed under the notion of *'izza'al*: anger, frustration, and disappointment that when it accumulates in the individual ultimately engenders poor health.

Abu Hassan is a very quiet man. His is the image of the man withdrawn into himself in the midst of a large and noisy family, sitting in his white *gallabiya* on the small *kanab* (little couch) in the hallway/living room. He frequently expresses his general content and gratefulness for what he has in life by the gesture of kissing his hand from the inside and outside several times. It was only through observing a number of arguments and fights within the family that I understood what he meant by the notion of *'izza'al*. In and after arguments underlying issues of pressure and tension often remain ultimately unsolved, which leads individuals to accumulate a growing sense of disappointment and unvoiced resentments. These build up to a pressing sense of *'izza'al*, which thus constitutes a pervasive feeling in individuals' lives beyond the limited instance of fighting and controversy. This feeling and its necessary oppression are closely connected to, and can be explained by, the notion of *katm,* which means to suppress feelings of discontent and disappointment. When a person experiences *'izza'al* and has to suppress (*yiktim*) his or her feelings and hopes, *'izza'al* consequently can be transformed into physical symptoms. A person who is unhappy about the way he is treated by others or by life in general is sometimes described as carrying unhappiness inside (*shāyil guwwāh*). The term *katm* suggests that *'iḍḍaghṭ* occurs in *al-nafs* (the person—see the introductory chapter), rather than the body or the mind.

This issue of *al-katm* illustrates a deeper aspect of health connected to my earlier discussion of *al-nafs* in the introductory chapter. The noun *katm* is derived from the root *ka-ta-ma*, which is used primarily to mean blocking the breath. The Arabic term for breath is *nafas*, which shares the same root with the word *nafs* or the person. I argue that the connection between *'izza'al* and *katm* means that *'iḍḍaghṭ* is perceived as a result of oppression of daily life, which I will discuss in the end of this chapter.

Feelings of *'izza'al* in Abu Hassan's family largely originated in their economic crises which started in the early 1980s when Abu Hassan and the eldest son, Hassan, were holding more profitable and stable employment. The family owned a car, and a van, which they rented out. Um Hassan describes those good days with the remark that they used to have a picnic every other week. A few years later Abu Hassan retired from work, and Ahmad and his younger brothers one after the other lost their jobs. The short-term jobs, which they had afterwards, are much less rewarding compared to the ever-rising cost of living. It was at this point that Abu Hassan fell ill for the first time. Around the same time the family had to accept a marriage proposal for one of the daughters where the future husband would move in with the family rather than provide a separate apartment for himself and his new wife, as is the common custom. The other daughter was widowed in the same time period and her in-laws sent her back to her father's house. It was at this point that spatial pressure was added to other pressures in the family's life. The oldest son, Nasser, who still lives with his parents because he cannot afford to marry and set up his own household, once remarked: "this is exactly what caused my father to get sick, because many people pressured him to accept my sister back. It is not only my sister, we are all a pressure to my father in this house, look at how many we are and how many problems we created in his life." Then, he added with a cynical laugh: "an entire government could get *'iḍḍaghṭ* under such circumstances . . . my father had a lot of *'izza'al* . . . he could not do anything but hide it." In a similar context looking dismayed yet maintaining his calm smile, Abu Hassan noted: "the best thing in this case is to pray to God, and put even more trust in him."

Abu Hassan is a very disciplined patient and shows great respect for his doctors' advice. When talking about his illness and treatment he always made a point of pronouncing the foreign names of his medicines correctly as he had learned some English while working in a large oil company in the 1960s. He felt that he had in such ways acquired a basic familiarity with the workings of aspects of a different type of knowledge and he was thus partaking in the process of his treatment. Nevertheless, he regards these medicines as useless without his reading of the Quran, which he does regularly: "it makes me calm and peaceful . . . that's what eventually counts, refuge in God." Abu Hassan rarely leaves the apartment and explains that: "my illness made it too difficult for me to go up and down the stairs." He even gave up attending the Friday prayers in the mosque. When he feels pain, family members call a physician neighbor to examine their father in his home. His sons and daughters buy his medication.

Um Hassan also has *'iḍḍaghṭ*, yet this is not her main problem. In general, she is more outspoken about her pains than her husband. Today, she carries most of the responsibility in the family and enjoys the authority that comes with that. Before Abu Hassan fell ill, things were very different. Um Hassan runs every detail of the household and aspects of the individual members' lives as well. Um Hassan finished six years of elementary school and thus has basic reading and writing skills, though rarely has a chance to use them. She is economically dependent on her husband and sons. The husband and the son are in turn socially dependent on her. She emphasizes that she "hosts" all her children (all along or after their return) in the house that she originally rented and furnished, which is true and none of them would argue with her about this. They emphasize their wish to be able to afford their own households. Simultaneously, they acknowledge the benefits of sharing the living costs. This allows each one to live cheaper and accumulate more for their individual futures, and even more so provides invaluable emotional support. The large sharing household, however, comes with its shadow of tension arising in the overcrowded space. Nevertheless, everyone agrees on the common saying reminiscent of Dr. Fawzi's notion of sharing: "*Lu'ma haniyya tikaffi miyya*" (one enjoyable morsel is enough for a hundred).

Um Hassan suffers from a possibly larger variety of illnesses and ailments than her husband does. She would often jokingly say to me: "I am a moving hospital, why don't you write only about me . . . they will give you a whole doctorate degree straight away when you tell them my story." She has rheumatic arthritis, diabetes, gastric and colon ulcers in addition to *'iḍḍaghṭ*. Nevertheless, she has never claimed the sick role as her husband has. She keeps moaning with pain whenever she does or says something. Unlike her husband she cannot afford the "sick role" in the house but runs frequent errands to secure food or other items on sale for the family or to make the obligatory visits to relatives to maintain valuable family ties. Despite all this her husband and sons would maintain that *'iḍḍaghṭ* is a male disease as it affects those who "think and work hard." They would argue that men are stronger than women, and for that reason they work harder. As I raised the issue of the immense strength required for multiple pregnancies Abu Hassan said: "that is the strength of Allah, not women."

Um Hassan is a disciplined patient and follows the physicians' advice. She further commands a considerable knowledge about health and disease, which she has accumulated from different sources such as herbalists, spiritual healers, doctors, and relatives and friends. Furthermore, she is an ardent fan of TV where she always pays close attention to health-related topics. Upon the advice of her doctor Um Hassan worked hard to lose fifteen kilograms but still thinks she remains somewhat overweight. She keeps a variety of herbs in the house, which she would readily recommend to me whenever I complained of some pain or cold. Nevertheless, she is always cautious to say that these herbs also need to be taken in ways to conform or harmonize with doctors' advice.

Um Hassan also attributes prominence to *'izza'al* with regard to her physical state. She describes *'izza'al* associated with the death of her younger sister about fifteen years ago as a starting point for some of her ailments. She recognises a direct connection between *'iḍḍaghṭ* and what she calls *'aṣabiyya* (nervousness) or *narfaza* (also a form of nervousness). Like *'izza'al*, *narfaza* generally means anger but denotes temporary and repetitive outbreaks of anger and high temper in everyday encounters. Um Hassan is considered *'assabiyya*, or nervous, by her family. She often gets angry and hurls, at times fierce, verbal abuse at family members. The latter for the most part avoid confrontations with her. In Um Hassan's explanatory scheme *narfaza* is directly related to *'izza'al*, especially with regard to poverty. She draws a correlation between the category of *al-ghalābah*, or those poor people whose life is embittered by hardship and frustration and subsequently are susceptible to *'izza'al*. *Al-ghalābah* in this sense is more often used to refer to those yet worse off than oneself, and only in more desperate situations would she refer to her own family as *al-ghalābah*.

CONCLUSION

Medical anthropologists have long discussed diseases as being deeply integrated into the structure of society. Some distinguish between the concept of "disease" and the concepts of "illness" and "sickness." Disease is a biological phenomenon, while the latter two concepts are social processes responsible for shaping individual and collective experiences (Frankenberg 1980; Young 1982; see also Lock and Gordon 1988). According to Young (1982) disease "refers to abnormalities in the structure and/or function of organs and organ systems; pathological states whether or not they are culturally recognised; the arena of the biomedical model" (Young 1982: 270). In contrast, illness "refers to a person's perceptions and experiences of certain socially devalued states including, but not limited to, disease" (*ibid.*).

These definitions are strongly relevant, although not totally adequate for my analysis of *'iḍḍaghṭ*. The concept of disease does not account for the possibility that other models of therapy have biophysical perspectives to describe biological malfunctions. Byron Good (1995), for example, notes that underlying this problem are difficulties of translating cultural concepts into biomedical ones. Byron Good (1995), based on his research on heart distress in Iran, confirms that cultural concepts about the physical aspects of disease are incorporated into "a complex set of semiotic relationships" that are not limited to the referential relation of sign to its physiological source" (*ibid*: 93) as represented in biomedicine.[1] In other words, the conceptual space of the "biophysical" can also be part of a cultural universe that connects it to the area of the individual consciousness (illness) and social experience (sickness) in a multitude of ways that is hardly translatable into purely bioscientific terms.

Also, underlying this problem is the reliance of early anthropological writings on the biomedical assumptions that separate the body and the mind, as implied in the distinction between "disease" and "illness." More recently this perspective has been reconsidered and analyzed as a particular rather than universalistic approach to the human health. Studies which are implicitly based on such biomedical assumptions were further criticized for their cultural bias toward modern biomedicine and for employing double standards when evaluating treatment effects (Lewis 1993a). "Double standards," Lewis notes, "go unrecognized in our own actions." (*ibid*: 192). In the case of biomedicine, therapeutic effects are taken for granted, once believed, and hardly questioned. Conversely, speaking about those who try to understand how nonwestern therapies work, Lewis notes,

> We are too ready to credit the mysterious powers of psychological and psychosomatic forces when the cases come from distant places and are about Aborigines or Africans. The readiness goes with a certain romanticism about exotic people and a set of attitudes or beliefs attributing emotional lability or oddness to other people, especially those called primitive, simple, or oriental (*ibid*: 193).

Furthermore, states of health, illness, as well as experience of pain have been recently viewed as lived by a "mindful body" (Scheper-Hughes and Lock 1987). The biophysical constitution of the body was reconsidered in the context of Foucault's philosophy, which views the modern biotechnologies as techniques of power and social control. In this perspective, the body provides the modern forms of the individual body-self, the symbols used in constructing the relations between nature, society, and culture, as well as the techniques for social and political control. This view now holds true for many anthropologists not only in theoretical terms but in practical ones, where conventional biomedical practice is seen "as to virtually assure inadequate diagnosis and unsuccessful treatment" (Kleinman et. al. 1994: 9).

The above situations display a rich pool of explanatory schemes where the present social and economic circumstances in Cairo are perceived by the sufferers from *'iḍḍaghṭ* as having adverse effects on the health of the city population. They are perceived as contributing to raising the blood pressure via two main routes: social pressures mediated by emotions with harmful effects, and pollution. Both routes originate in the social relations that organise and produce the individual bodies. The body is firmly interwoven with the social and economic environments through the mediating force of emotions. Morsy's (1980) insights on the beliefs about the body here gain support. Based on her research in the Egyptian Delta she concludes that among the members of the community "the proper functioning of the body is not independent of its surroundings" (*ibid.*: 92). Biomedicine also views the body in relation to its social and ecological environments. In practice, however, the dominant approach is to "investigate disease as an individual matter, concentrating on the person and the body rather than the social setting" (Lewis 1993b: 88). Furthermore, biomedicine excludes the causes of pain engendered by the emotions and which form strong connections between the mind and the body. This is especially true in the case of chronic pain connected with high blood pressure as Kleinman et al. (1994) argue that the concept of chronic pain is

> so poorly defined that [its] syndromes lack official status within biomedical taxonomy. The American Psychiatric Association's *DSM-III* category of "Psychogenic Pain"—subsequently dropped in *DSM-III-R*—was unacceptable because physicians and psychologists find relatively few cases of pain in which the etiology is clearly and solely psychological, what one finds is a profusion of discrete conditions—low back pain, chest pain (without heart or lung pathology), functioning bowel syndrome, headaches, and so on—without agreement on a unifying rubric (*ibid.*: 4).

Despite the problems with the anthropological definitions of disease and illness noted above, the concept of sickness remains useful to discuss the problem of *'iḍḍaghṭ*. I hold that this concept helps in analyzing the individual body and consciousness, as well as the collective activities carried out to overcome various socially devalued states of being, as belonging to one interactive field. In the words of Young (1982) *sickness* refers to processes where

> worrisome behavioral and biological signs, particularly ones originating in disease, are given socially recognized meanings, i.e. they are made into symptoms and socially significant outcomes. In short, sickness is "*a process for socializing disease and illness*" (emphasis in original) (*ibid.*).

This distinction rests upon the generally accepted premise that "every culture has rules for translating signs into symptoms, for linking symptomatologies to aetiologies and interventions, and for using the evidence provided by interventions to confirm translations and legitimize outcomes" (*ibid.*). *'Iḍḍhaghṭ* is a sickness constructed by using biomedical and humoral Islamic concepts and methods. It is a socialized disease in a double sense. First, its meanings are dialectically linked to social processes and symbols deeply integrated into the structure of society. Its symptoms are explained by factors with social origins, and simultaneously used to describe social relations. Second, the paths that people follow to cope with *'iḍḍaghṭ* are associated with a field of meanings produced by various social institutions including the medical enterprise, the mass media, religion, and the family. It is the collective product of these institutions that formulates what I call the "social discourse on *'iḍḍaghṭ*."

Scheper-Hughes and Lock (1987) formulate the concept of sickness in relation to discourse in language in a way more relevant than the above definition by Young. They argue that

> Sickness is not just an isolated event, nor an unfortunate brush with nature. It is a form of communication—the language of the organs—through which nature, society, and culture speak simultaneously. The individual body should be seen as the most immediate, the proximate terrain where social truths and social contradictions are played out, as well as a locus of personal and social resistance, creativity, and struggle (*ibid.*: 31).

The narratives above show that the sickness of *'iḍḍaghṭ* is felt in Cairo not only in the individual body but also in aspects characterizing life as a whole. As such, the meanings located in this terrain express processes, feelings, events, and experiences that transcend the pure physical understandings of the disease (see Good 1977; Blumhagen 1980). High blood pressure is a sign for the medicalization of social life in Cairo. It is a process where the adverse effects of the economic privatization followed by the government starting from the mid-1970s are constructed as treatable by pills for high blood pressure. But *'iḍḍaghṭ* does have the meaning of high blood pressure. In the words of Blumhagen (1980) who did his research on mainstream urban America, *'iḍḍaghṭ* in Cairo has become a "folk illness with a biomedical name." In other words, upon the deployment of the concept of high blood pressure, a discourse has been set to define the various meanings in terms specific to Egypt's historical culture, meanings that best express the society's structural relations of power, contradictions, and ambivalences.

The physicians who are ill with *'iḍḍaghṭ* offer multiple voices in their explanations of their illness, including the conventional models they received at school. The role of their cultural background in accounting for the socio-economic circumstances specific to the environment of Cairo is evident in their emphasis on the relevance of the social pressures in their lives. Their narratives illustrate the link between the professional and the popular models of interpretation, which are obviously inspired by the linguistic forms that shape health experience. My argument is that both kinds of models are encompassed and in a continuous process of interaction that leads into a dynamic field of interpretation and therapy responsible for producing the current phenomenon of *'iḍḍaghṭ*.

All the persons included evaluate the therapies they receive at clinics as good for treating only one aspect of suffering. When they refer to therapies such as biomedical pills they consider them as *musakkināt*, or the means to suppress their physical pains originating in their family relations or their position in surrounding social and economic environments. The patients suffering from *'iḍḍaghṭ* are not concerned with the series of causes and effects that may take place inside the body, which the physicians often reiterate in their talks in the mass media or during their consultations with their patients. It is not that patients refute physicians' theories or actively reject particular medicines. This is not their major concern or field of inquiry. Their complaints are directly related to the oppressive conditions of their daily life.

Common to all the experiences above, environmental pollution adds another dimension to the outside pressures on each person's well-being. Abu Hassan further adds the element of noise as a problem both of the city at large and in his household in particular. Zaina mentions the contraceptive pill, which has profound implications for the theme of female sexuality and the notion of pollution. I argue that the semantics of *'iḍḍaghṭ* discussed above derive from biomedicine in addition to ideas rooted in Islamic and Greek humoral medicine. Byron Good (1995) notes that the theme of pollution is also mentioned in *al-Muqaddimah* by Ibn Khaldun, a classical scholar who lived in Cairo in the fourteenth century and whose work centered on the theme of the rise and decline of civilizations. Ibn Khaldun relied on notions of humoral medicine to make a connection between elements of the air, the energy, the spirit, and general health, all conceived as elements in the process of digestion that provided the basis for physiological and medical reasoning in Islamic medicine (B. Good 1995: 107–108). But none of the traditions involved in explaining *'iḍḍaghṭ* exists as a uniform or homogeneous system. Instead, various elements are presented as fragments, which gain meaning and coherence from the patients' experiences situated in the plural medical system. This coherence is temporally conditioned and contingent on the social and cultural circumstances surrounding the illness terms. The anthropological search for homogeneous isolated culture-bound concepts of illness is not feasible in the present world of coexisting, interacting, and changing health traditions.

'Iḍḍaghṭ is a chronic disease with no solution that any of the individuals included foresee. No single patient expressed hope of changing the settings responsible for producing this syndrome. They all, however, say they find relief by following certain combinations of therapeutic measures to cope with their pains. They hope that the therapeutic composites will at least help control the symptoms of *'iḍḍaghṭ* in their personal lives. The multiplicity of these measures thus expresses the manifold meanings of *'iḍḍaghṭ* and reflects a number of opposing domains useful in understanding the composition of the worldview producing the perceptions of *'iḍḍaghṭ*.

Most of the patients, along with the biomedical pills, take hibiscus, which is an herb widely used for its calming or cooling effects. Other patients mentioned cool showers as a therapeutic measure. These practices indicate that *'iḍḍaghṭ* falls into the class of hot ailments, which is an additional evidence of the presence of the classical notions of humoral medicine in Cairo today. Also, many respondents mentioned prayers as a coping measure. Next to its effect of coping with the illness, however, prayers are a reminder of a world of purity and justice as opposed to the unfair treatment characterizing the present world, as in the case of Dr. Fawzi. Connected to the theme of prayers is the notion of a glorious past for which all patients long. They mention that the present time is radically different from past times in the 1950s and 1960s. At that time, the city was more spacious, cleaner, and offered better food. Social relations during those times were also different; they were more intimate and less competitive than at the present time. Whether real or fictitious, this construction has been reiterated by innumerable people in Cairo in the context of their talk about *'iḍḍaghṭ* and other issues of relating to their oppressive daily life, evident in the theme of social pressures discussed above. Interestingly, not all those people suffer from the signs of *'iḍḍaghṭ*, but they all feel those signs and conditions which host the ailment in the air they breathe and the food they eat and which will become part of their bodies.

On the whole, high blood pressure is translated into *'iḍḍaghṭ*, which is formulated to express the life and culture of the people living in Cairo. The meanings of *'iḍḍaghṭ* cover areas wider than those covered by the parent biomedical concept. Although it is certainly a sign of the increasing medicalization of Egyptian society, it has nevertheless been appropriated and articulated in innumerable ways relevant to persons suffering from the pressures of modern life. Whether viewed as a biomedical category or a popular concept of sickness, *'iḍḍaghṭ* has become an integral part of the cultural scene of today's Cairo where its meanings are determined by the specific linguistic forms available to the imagination of those who suffer from it.

Finally, the discourse on *'iḍḍaghṭ* illustrates how the family and the social relations of society at large are implicated in the production of concepts of health and illness. It also illustrates the kind of social institutions involved in maintaining the plural character of health traditions. The next chapter will further illustrate how the perceptions of the body, health, illness, life and death are subjects of a national debate that involves the medical, religious, political, and legal institutions which, while striving to appropriate new biotechnologies, try to maintain the integrity of their social structure and the continuity of their traditions.

NOTES

1. Gilbert Lewis (1993b) arrives at a similar conclusion about the unfeasibility of connecting the system of diagnosis among the Gnau with the western biomedical diagnostic categories (*ibid*: 106–109).

4

Health and Wellness in Life and Death

This chapter examines debates focused on the morality of organ transplantation. I am concerned with how the notion of life discussed so far is constructed in contexts of society at large, and more particularly within different forms of social governance represented by the family, religion, and the state. In particular, I seek to describe and analyze these notions in contexts of opposed views on the morality of the controversial notion of brain death and technologies for transferring of body parts between different persons. I note that the participants in these debates are divided between those who support the new practices and those calling to adapt them to local traditions. My assumptions are as follows. Firstly, life technologies are advanced technical means for maintaining, altering, and improving conditions of life, health, illness, healing, and death. Their inherently materialistic approach to life and society is produced within market-oriented industries based on philosophical assumptions viewing social relations as links between things rather than mindful bodies endowed with tradition-bound rights and duties. Therefore, they stir debates focused on their moral ramifications everywhere. In the present context I assume that the opinions of each group of debaters are congruent with their respective social interests. On one side there are the proponents of the incoming technologies who more or less straightforwardly view them as scientific, and thus good, solutions for particular medical conditions. They would ultimately help in solving major health problems facing society as a whole. Furthermore, they are part of a moral mission closely related to the values of cooperation and virtues of altruism, which are immensely significant for social cohesion. The call to adopt these techniques is backed by the state, the mainstream medical establishment with evident connections with the global market, and particular religious authorities.

On the other hand there are interlocutors who view the new technologies relationally; they address issues of the body, the person, and community in this world and after death. They demonstrate that these concepts are original and central subjects to their long-held traditions shaped by both cooperative and conflictual relations of power rooted in different modes of life. They receive the proposed idea to "donate" bodies defined as brain-dead and body parts of living persons to others who need them to recover from otherwise incurable illnesses with extreme caution. Categories of the body and life in Egypt are extraordinarily precious, exceedingly intimate, and religiously sacred subjects.

Most interesting to my argument is the fact that the discourse on life is exacerbated because it is ultimately based on particular moral questions central to the society's entire political economic structure—the moral discourse discussed in the introduction. These debaters manage to use medical ideas to build far-reaching arguments of moral critique stemming from the body and reaching up to society's higher ideals of the good life. I believe that these views follow the interlocutors' political-economic interests; those who propagate the incoming techniques and concepts represent the mainstream medical establishment backed by the modernizing state and its favored representatives of religion. Their views are ultimately cultural elaborations of globalized commodities rooted in the capitalist market. The ones who are critical of them offer alternative ways to conceptualize life in terms of *al-nafs*, an otherworldly concept with profound implications for current social life including its mundane material and political struggles. I view this conceptualization as *life-surge*—an immortal force rooted in the notion of the soul or person as a morally laden motif pervading the society's traditions. I hold that the life-surge is manifested in the enthusiastic pursuit toward maintaining life as a holistic category with strong ethical significance. It consists of positive energies engaged in everyday life, of which death is an integral part. It aims at lifting various elements suspected of muddling the general sense of wellness and issues of growth, national pride, and continuity. Furthermore, it moderates between opposed forces of sin and virtue and thus speaks of a tension generated by unstable states of being characterizing social life in this world generally. Most interesting is that *al-nafs* is ultimately part of a discourse with an eschatological dimension aiming at protecting life in this world by constructing it as part of God as the ultimate goal of all morals.

I view the pro- and anti-donation arguments as constituents of a unified field operated by the plural health system and catalyzed by the notional life-surge rooted in *al-nafs* as a morally binding force. All kinds of views try to relate to traditions. The pro-donation argument however is a mechanical elaboration of globalized technologies into local traditional terms. The anti-donation arguments seek persuasion through the notion of *al-nafs* as a unifying capacity representing the social strife for a state of correctness within individual bodies living now and after death. These arguments are built around a core belief in Islam that different bodies are ultimately enlivened by *al-nafs-alwāḥida* (the one and only soul) of God—the original and *one* creator of the entire universe. In this sense organ transference between different bodies is situated within a tradition oriented to realize *ṣiḥḥa* (health) as a comprehensive state of moral coherence manufactured in contexts of the family, religion, and the state and profoundly affected by the dominant political economic structures of society.

The rest of this chapter consists of the following. First, I describe the social context within which the debates occur. I argue that it is composed of a "soft state," characterized by a hegemonic political economy of capitalistic market, increasingly marketized rules of life intruding into a continuing tradition and society marked by surviving different modes of production. The debate on brain death illustrates that the body is conceived as an aspect rather an antonym to the mind. I argue that *al-nafs* is an otherworldly notion remade as a tradition-based critical means to defend the interests of the underprivileged classes in an increasingly unjust society where the life of some is used to improve or prolong the life of some privileged others.

The debates therefore are handy in exploring the way the notions central to social life discussed in the previous chapters at local levels are reproduced in society-wide discourses involving the state and major institutions of religion and the law.

POLITICAL ECONOMY AND CONTINUED TRADITIONS

Viewed through the above ideas of praxis, tradition, and critical reason, the debates on the morality and legality of organ transplantation are a *discursive field of power* that enable different sections of society to speak about their lives in ways congruent with their interests. On one hand, there is the hegemonic political economic system led by the state and causing deep social schisms. On the other there is a reaction led by the local traditions tied partly to the penetrative system but articulated in differing terms rooted in modes of production operating in the undocumented spheres of life. Included for example is small commodity production well documented in the studies of the informal (AbdelFadil 2011). The rest of this chapter relays how this reaction takes place.

Health care practices in Cairo operate within contexts of the family, the local community, and society at large. My argument so far is that the ways health resources are utilized and evaluated ultimately form an index of a plural system concerned not merely with curing physical diseases but with the very general state of well-being represented by life as an original human attribute deeply associated with a strong sense of morality. In chapter 1 the moral argument is represented in psychiatry and spiritual healing. In chapter 2 it is represented by the obligations between emotional ties and family members. In chapter 3 almost all the explanations of *'iḍḍaghṭ* are about the moral aspects of contemporary life in Cairo characterized by *dughūṭ alḥayaah* (life pressures) medicated by the traditionally held notion of *al-nafs*. These pressures affect not merely physical health. More profoundly, they damage the local *sense of wellness* conceived in a holistic fashion as an optimum state of balance characterizing the body. In other words, wellness is essentially an attribute of persons living in morally defined environments mediated through the notion of *al-nafs* as a tradition-bound space adapted to perform a moral critique of deteriorating life conditions.

The Egyptian modes of life are deeply rooted in history. This is why the issues discussed hitherto illustrate that the individuals who are viewed and treated as bodies under the influence of biomedicine act as persons inseparable from long-lived communal relationships. Forces discussed under the local term of *ḍughūṭ al-ḥayāh* for example illustrate that biomedical constructions ultimately operate within larger plural systems that reproduce anew the notion of *'iḍḍaghṭ* as a traditional social category. It represents not merely the physical conditions that are recognized from the biomedical perspective, but more profoundly the various ways people *feel*, *evaluate*, and *act on* their sufferings from multiple socioeconomic, political, and emotional *dūghūṭ* (pressures) rather than the singular *ḍḍaghṭ* (pressure) articulated in physical terms. My argument is that *'iḍḍaghṭ* is essentially a notion produced in a large process of *cultural critique* based on emotions, feelings, and ideas rooted in the local traditions geared to evaluating general conditions of life. I would further argue that it is a manifestation of a *social crisis* exemplified by the increasingly unbearable circumstances and conditions impinging on people's lives traditionally perceived as something that should be kept in good balance. Biomedicine, of course, contributes to this crisis because it assists in constructing the current realities in apparently neutral terms while in practice it is deeply rooted in the dominant globalized market. Within the context of neoliberal economics it shares many of this system's ideological premises—it is a predominantly materialistic, individual-based, profit-maximizing, class-biased enterprise.

Similarly, the ideas circulated in the debates on organ transplantation are produced within general discourses on wellness conceived as a general whole aspect essential to life in this world and after death. Underlying the participants' opinions are notions and sensibilities tightly connected to the discourses on life including, most significantly, the notion of *al-nafs*, which I view as the cultural equivalent of what some call the "mindful body" (cf. Scheper-Hughes and Lock 1987) equipped with "multi-sensory modes of attention" that enable it to "be-in-the-world" (Csordas 1993). I prefer the notion of *al-nafs* over that of the body because it departs from the purely materialistic approaches to life characteristic of the now-particularistic modern biomedicine. In addition, *al-nafs* is pervaded by a sense of morality. Crucial to this chapter is that *al-nafs* is a cultural fact pointing to an immortal capacity; it is believed to stay alive after the body perishes. During life it constantly speaks to people and affects their decisions. After death it remains present; it receives gifts in the form of immolations, graveyard visits, and offerings to the poor. Most interesting is that after death *al-nafs* remains as an active agent in social relations among the living through the notion of pain.

Organ transplantations are complex operations, not only technically but also socially, morally, and politically. They relate to issues of social struggle fuelled by perceived social injustice. They offer an opportunity to further explore the way the plural health system is linked to social relations of power in contexts of society, the state, law, and religion. In particular, they help identify how the notions of human subjects are variously *configured* in life and death. I assume that life is essentially another expression of the notion of *al-nafs* manifest through the body although not totally dependent on it.

As mentioned earlier, plural health resources can be viewed as a general discourse concerned with representing as well as *feeling* different manifestations of life not simply as static conditions of health and illness but as complex and dynamic fields constituted by combinations of circumstances that are not simply embodied but *ensouled.*

The issue of *al-nafs* is intriguing for another reason. It is not limited by birth and death. Those who debate organ donation, for example, believe that *al-nafs* exists before birth and stays after death. This difference gives the views of life under consideration specific meanings of a field consisting of diverse *states of being* driven by what I call *life-surge*; *a boundless, never-ending capacity inducing various kinds of action in and through others even when the body it has once enlivened is dead. Al-nafs* is able to assuming various kinds and forms and magnitudes of wellness and pain independent of the body. For example, *al-nafs* is believed to suffer for not fulfilling a promise it has once made to others or to God. It is relieved from suffering when that promise is fulfilled on its behalf by one of its descendants. Therefore, *al-nafs* is agentive in the social sense of the term. These attributes are minutely interlaced with issues of pain and unwellness that may develop into recognized illnesses, imbalance, or death.

In practice, the hegemonic market economy in Egypt contributes to the transformation of medical services into a commodity aiming at curing rather than healing socially rooted complaints. The phrase that "medical care has become *tigārah*" (mere business) has been a household term in Cairo throughout recent decades. It is in this context that life technologies are perceived as emblematic for issues of the objectification of social life, including, of course, life and the body. In addition, I think these technologies intensified an already existing sense of fragmentation due to the view of the body as a breakable, atomistic material entity owned by discrete individuals rather than morally laden persons or *ashkhāṣ* (sing. *shakhṣ*) belonging to larger communities. I argue that the debates under consideration are not about the body *per se*. They are ultimately about much deeper social disparities of moral character between the haves and the have-nots. I argue that this sense is ultimately linked to the fact that society has been severely divided; on the one side, there are those individuals who managed to make fortunes in a relatively short period starting with the liberalization of the market. On the other side, tens of millions have been impoverished or at least did not benefit to the same extent (see Amin 1988). In either case, commentators have explained deepening divisions as resulting from corruption associated with excessive marketization of public resources that formerly were run for the benefit of the whole society.

This context, locally described by critics as "malformed economy" (*iqtiṣād mushawwah*), is driven by greedy capitalists who also managed to control the state apparatus. This economy transformed many significant aspects of social life. Those who managed to profit very quickly were assisted by representatives of corrupt governments that used low-intensity democracy to cover up authoritarian rulers who "weaseled" their way to maximize their individual gains. These few used various legal tricks devised by "legal tailors" (*tarziyyit al-qawānīn*, as noted earlier in the study) to alter existing codes to fit their goals. "Dubious" is the term that best describes this situation and the resulting sense of compromised safety in Cairo not only about one's possessions but also about one's own body. This sense of suspicion and doubt has infiltrated the public imagery and appeared in major social representations such as films,[1] books,[2] and political commentary to which the debates discussed here belong.

Organ transplants belong to a globalized industry. The state and the world system are therefore essential categories for their analysis. In local contexts, however, they take up meanings unique to the local traditions and social structures. In contemporary societies perceptions, notions, and values are hardly, if ever, uniform or harmonious. I view the debates as a cultural sphere constructed in terms of the plural health system noted above. I hold that this system results from multiple modes of production characterizing social and economic life in the country. In the face of the economic transformation summarized above this plurality has been reduced under the influence of marketization and concomitant biomedicalization. Certain aspects of *al-nafs* that occur in the course of the debate including the ideas of growth, pain, and immortality are essential to the traditions responding to the new technologies.

I believe these ideas belong to modes of socioeconomic life that are both engaged and distant from the dominant capitalistic mode. They have also been diversified internally due to uneven developments; social formations within nation-states for example may include elements of what may be analytically regarded as different modes of production. The material elements included in these modes are inseparable from the ways they are socially organized as well as the ways these organizations are perceived, conceptualized, and felt, or symbolically represented in accordance to local norms, values, and discourses. The latter category of discourse includes practice mediating material and immaterial aspects of life; it provides grounds upon which principles of social organization are debated, evaluated, and reconstructed. In modern society discourses are produced by central institutions through unified legal and ethical codes. The latter however are either totally or partly rooted in the shared traditions of the communities and societies concerned, a fact that results in more intense debates and conflicts between and within traditions. These conflicts yield diverse practical interpretations of traditions.

The previous interpretations of traditional therapeutic methods (chapter 1) are good examples. Tradition ultimately refers to fields of reasoning and thinking linked to practical life and "transcending the limitations of what had hitherto been reasoned in that tradition [which] is true of modern physics as of medieval logic" (MacIntyre 1984: 222). I think this transcendence results from critical thinking performed by practical reason in quest for solutions of problems threatening life or safety.

The current debates take place in contexts of the state and law. The latter is a strategic means used to destroy old options and create new ones. The call to adopt the new technologies belongs to this same practice. These are based on understandings and moral considerations of human life essentially different from the ones sustained by the local traditions. Ideally, the state is a sovereign body that regards the local population as equal citizens subjected to well-defined rights and duties. It uses the law for "creating conditions in which equal citizens can do certain things as 'free agents'" (Asad 1992: 336). This description does not apply to the state in Egypt that has evidently fallen short of providing necessary ideological and administrative conditions of law-regulated institutions. This failure is most obvious in the relative absence of legislation and implementation of the rules and legal codes to regulate various kinds of practices relating to its subjects' lives, including of course those relating to life technologies.

Next to corruption associated with its withdrawal from almost all public services as discussed earlier, the state showed excessive amounts of laxity in enforcing the law equally on all subjects. It uses brutal force against citizens who protest its power. Furthermore, the state has been very dependent and colluded with foreign political and economic powers for the benefit of its representatives and local and international capitalists. The implications of such power for the debates on organ transplantation are immense; the surgeries are felt to be occurring in contexts that are ultimately influenced by the state of corruption characterizing state and society as a whole. In some sense, they occur in a sick atmosphere similar to that engendering *'iḍḍaghṭ* and thus should be resisted.

This resistance relies on a continuing tradition. Here the plural health system of Cairo participates in a multivocal way represented by different institutions that continue to represent social struggles despite, or possibly because of, their inclusion under the umbrella of the nation-state that is supposed to represent them all. In the debates that follow, I am not concerned with supporting particular positions against others. My concern is with the ways the participants diversely use the categories offered by the plural system of health care to describe their opinions. More particular, I am concerned with exploring how the notions of the body, life, wellness, and death underlying their arguments are used relationally. Later in this chapter I will discuss the implications of these concepts for the power structure of society.

INSTITUTIONALIZED DISCOURSE

All the institutions participating in the debate are supposed to be connected and regulated by the state. In practice, however, they are not univocal. Each of them has different and at times conflicting views. Further, some institutions like religion have representatives who are almost completely independent of the state. Medical care also shows some resistance to state authority. The disagreements however are not on the legitimacy of the state. They are about the rules of power practices. In brief, the issue of legalizing organ transference is evidently sponsored by the state and the medical enterprise. It is an integral part of the macro transformation taking place in the whole country and heading toward privatizing the economic system and along with it many aspects of social life including traditional views and laws about the body. My argument is that much of this power is opposed by what I suggested to call tradition-rooted life-surge—its views of the body, wellness, and health and illness during life and after death. Life-surge is ultimately rooted in this world and its social struggles.

One major institution participating in the debates is al-Azhar, the millennial mosque and school of the Foundations of Religion (*'usūl al-dīn*), Islamic Jurisprudence (*al-Sharī'a)* and Arabic Language. Al-Azhar has always been integrated into everyday life of modern society. For the last fifty years it has been developed into a modern institution run according to standard bureaucracy overseeing its whole activities. The school gave rise to a university including faculties of engineering, agriculture, and most relevant for the present context, medicine. Significantly, al-Azhar continues to maintain and develop long-standing organizations for religious services and, research, the most important of which is the Islamic Assembly of Researches, responsible for issuing religious opinions or advice (*fatwas*), which play major roles in the debates under consideration as well as many other issues and controversies. This institution, therefore, represents an important modernized traditional institution so to speak. Since the 1950s it has been annexed by the state. Its grand Imam has since then been appointed by the country's president. But that did not mean the institution has become totally uniform; many of the sheikhs representing views differing from the grand Imam receded to less prominent positions but continued to immensely influence the public. Some of these belong to the popular group of the Muslim Brotherhood. It is noteworthy that important figures from this group have adamantly resisted the new technologies.

The second government-allied religious institution that plays an important role in these debates is the Department of *al-'iftā'* (the process of issuing *fatwas*, or religious scholarly opinions). The Mufti of the Republic of Egypt, Imam Nasr Farid Wassel, heads this institution. The lines separating al-Azhar and the Department of *al-'iftā'* are not always clear. In the case of organ transplantation, however, the two institutions collaborated in producing one major *fatwa*. Parallel to these government-allied institutions and actors the debates include other interlocutors who represent popular Islam, such as Sheikh Muhammad Mitawalli al-Sha'raawi, who is also a graduate of al-Azhar, as mentioned above. Al-Sha'raawi is seen as an independent scholar in these debates. In the words of one Member of Parliament, the sheikh "has his freedom," while others, such as the Grand Imam and the Muftis do not. The latter are ultimately "government Muftis," according to a Member of Parliament writing for the weekly *al-Dustour* (27.11.1996).

The third institution involved in the debates is the doctors' syndicate represented by its head, Dr. Hamdi al-Sayyid. Representing the professional organization of medical science, Dr. al-Sayyid calls for unconditional acceptance of the new life technologies. The modernist science-based ideas of Dr. al-Sayyid however face strong resistance led by other doctors in his organization who have been resisting the new technologies. This institution, like many others that are ideally supposed to represent civil society, has been penetrated by the state power. That intervention never meant the end of opposed views.

The fourth institution of significant influence is the media. However, this is almost totally controlled by the state. It operates very well to maintain the regime's low-intensity democracy. The media, however, is keen to publish opposing views. It also benefits from the debate; it provides a sensual subject that attracts readership. The media therefore is predominantly an arm for the mother institution of the market.

The overwhelming authority of the state is evident in the fact that all the interlocutors generally affirm that their ultimate goal is to realize the common good of society and that they are guided by sets of ideals and cultural rules that would lead to the prosperity of the whole society. Furthermore, on the specific question of organ donation, most of them would agree on the noble ideals underlying these acts including their contribution to solidarity between family members as well as citizens of the same society. All these aims are clearly central to the modern state's mission. Disagreements occur upon dealing with the practical sides of organ transplantation, which is essentially what these therapies are all about. In practice, the above supposedly "shared ideas and feelings" are linked to what can be called *strategies* of different parties; their generally envisaged plans on how to realize their socioeconomic goals. The result of the interaction between these strategies is what I call *discourse* on organ transplantation. In the context of state policy this discourse is ultimately about power, whether this is sought for enabling or disabling the population concerned. For the "law is neither a transcendent principle of justice, nor an overarching framework of society" (Asad 1992: 335). It is part of the state's strategy to achieve control over the population through destroying its old laws and creating new ones that serve its power (*ibid*). These debates therefore shed light on some aspects of these strategies as they describe how the debaters *live* or at least how they feel and think their lives ought to be lived. Central to my argument is the idea that their ideas and feelings are conditioned by the concept of *al-nafs.* The latter constitutes many of the incentives to resist central power based on traditional views of justice and moderation that are linked to the notion of wellness of the individual and collective sense of the term.

In a sense, the discourse is like a *game* between the debaters' ideologies. Most notably there are the assumptions of modern biomedicine that are rooted in globalized multibillion-dollar pharmaceutical industries and supposedly aimed at preserving and promoting conditions for a better life. These, however, are inserted within a new sociocultural universe aiming at relevant achievements but oriented toward larger and more complex moral questions posed by and within local struggles.

The debaters are divided around these questions in ways reminiscent of the major social divisions created by the market economy. The first question for which the debaters strive to establish an answer is whether there should be a law accepting and regulating the new technologies. And if there will be, what are the social and ethical principles it should rest upon? Who should be allowed to donate organs and who should receive the donations? Could people be allowed to sell and buy organs? In all cases, who should have authority over the body? Are they the persons who live in those bodies, or their families? Should doctors be authorized to conduct these operations independent of state regulations? All these questions are familiar ones and have been described as having been discussed in many other societies.[3] In Cairo they have taken on a new life as the following discussion shows.

THE DEBATE

These debates were triggered by a group of interlocutors who have been urging society to accept the ideas of transplantations and to encourage all to perform what they call "organ donation" (*tabarru' bi al'ḍā*). They are mostly physicians who occupy official positions in the state and/or the National Democratic Party, which was in power for thirty years. They have sought to spread ideas into the public allowing the transference of organs from both patients called "brain dead" and those who are living and ready to "donate" one of their organs to others who have been chronically diseased by an incurable pain that might also threaten their life. The donors may then be compensated in material or immaterial forms. The donation enthusiasts, however, remain silent about this last idea of compensation. This group's argument is actually more or less a cultural elaboration on globalized life technologies known to be rooted in biochemical sciences, and oriented toward professional success linked to material profit in the market economy. The leading figures of this group do have a moralistic message. However, it is essentially the same standardized message focused on the altruistic values of organ donation, national needs, and scientific advancement. It is not difficult to figure that much of what they propagate is literal translations of familiar globalized clichés on "organ donation" initially launched in the United States before spreading in the rest of the world. These objectives are phrased using local cultural terms that are ready to refute (refute what?) on two grounds. First is their irrelevance to the major health challenges that Egypt faces. Second, and most significant, is the Egyptian health tradition characterized by a different approach to life and wellness rather than the body and illness.

Most prominent among the people who try to promote organ transplantation is the head of the doctor's syndicate, Dr. Hamdi al-Sayyid, who is quoted as saying:

> Egypt was once a leading and pioneering country. It led the Islamic world to adopt reasons for progress and civilization and developing Islamic thought in a way congruent with the scientific knowledge available at the time. But unfortunately, we regressed more and more as a result of a conspiracy, and ideas alien to Islamic thought (*al-Ahrām* 18.11.1995).

Furthermore, for Dr. al-Sayyid blocking the process of issuing a law that facilitates organ transplantation means hindering the moral mission of science. Accompanying this enthusiasm about science is a strong moral sense about the "many patients who will have no hope of recovery." Those who are opposed to organ transplantation, the doctor's argument goes on, "should be morally accountable before future generations" (*ibid*). The call for the adoption of organ transplantation is associated with a strong nationalist rhetoric, which is phrased in bodily terms. The economy of Egypt will be "suffocated because the government would have to spend great amounts of money on patients who would have to seek these therapies abroad" (*al-Akhbar* 10.2.1996).

Dr. al-Sayyid compares Egypt to other countries that have long permitted organ transplantation. He regrets that in countries such as Saudi Arabia, which became modernized long after Egypt, medicine is far more advanced. There, according to the physician, scientists proudly contribute to international medical research, whereas in Egypt,

> we are still weeping and licking our wounds and mourning over our misfortune while facing inflexibility and backwardness, and rigid ways of thinking about the definition of death since the days of the four Imams (*ibid*).

Some pro-state religious authorities help pro-donation physicians translate medical concepts into ones relevant to Islamic traditions. It is hoped that the latter will produce a *fatwa* to promote the physicians' authority over the body and render the consent of other parties such as the deceased's family members unnecessary (*al-Ahram* 10.6.1996). They define the notion of brain death in ways reminiscent of standardized definitions circulated in a wide variety of medical literature like the one produced by the Harvard Ad Hoc Committee on Brain Death. The doctors spend no special effort to translate this concept into local tradition. Their assumption seems to be that the public should automatically accept such medical concepts. This presumption is most notable especially when carried by professionals representing biomedicine, the most hegemonic system of therapy at both local and global levels. The local cultural introduction so to speak is performed by the Grand Imam of al-Azhar, and another major Imam called Yousuf al-Qradawi who is a well-known theologian and has been working as Head of the International Union of Muslim Scholars. He is also Egyptian and a graduate of al-Azhar. The two scholars argue that the body is a property given by God to humans to live by it and who are thus authorized to dispose of it. The two debaters openly urge everyone to support the doctors' call to legally accept brain death as a conclusive and absolute death after which human organs can be transferred to the bodies of other people to save their lives (*Almasry-Alyoum* 13.3.2009).[4]

The enthusiasm of the physicians and the support of the Imams are met by the pessimism, suspicion, and fear of other physicians, religious figures, and newspaper columnists. These express their distrust of the government and the medical establishment. I would argue that, in principle, these interlocutors are not essentially different from those who promote the practices of organ transplantation. As Moosa (1999) suggests, their knowledge, "namely medical and juristic, share the same moral and epistemological taxonomy" because they belong, or at very least, are speaking, meaning having to articulate their thoughts, in terms offered by the same tradition. Furthermore, they all show great inspiration from the same ideals, such as the notion of progress, the superiority of the social body over the individual body. However, they occupy different ideological positions within society and thus are aware of different political strategies and projects.

Those who resist Dr. al-Sayyid's call do not challenge the need to advance science or solve its health problems. These are also among their central concerns. Their contention occurs normally from their traditional understanding of the body and body parts as moral issues. A careful reading of the opinions of those debaters reveals that they are only apparently opposed to the new techniques. In essence, they are in support of the ideas. Their issue is that they situate the new surgeries within their own traditional paradigms on the body, that they treat in a relational manner in the midst of moral meanings of life, wellness, health, and death.

Most crucially, opponents of brain death insist that the meanings of notions of life, wellness, health, and death derive from the different ways they are *experienced* and *felt* by the individuals involved within their communities. These understandings, therefore, are relevant to the central question of this chapter in ways much more interesting than the biomedical ones noted above. The latter are ultimately rooted in local cultures that have been universalized by means of the market economy. Eventually they have infiltrated local worldviews. Nevertheless, these continue to be driven by localized structural forces that are best understood if studied in their own terms and within their specific forms of governance represented in the present context by the family, religion, and the state.

BRAIN DEATH

First, the anti-donation debaters tend to focus on beliefs and ideas deriving from the local traditions that also include biomedicine in the ways it has thus far been practiced in the country. This is nowhere clear as in the case of brain death. They would continue to hold to the traditional definition of death. In a conference held specifically to discuss the notion of brain death, the participants rejected the concept and reaffirmed the already existing definition of death, approved by the religious authorities. According to this definition, death occurs upon "the *departure* of the spirit from the body, the complete cessation of all organs, and coldness of the body. The spirit is the force which prevents the decomposition and rotting of the body" (*al-Ahram* 11.6.1996—emphasis added).

A prominent debater in this context is Dr. Safwat Lutfi, a physician and professor of anesthesiology at the Central Hospital and Medical School of Qasr al-Aini. "These are not purely medical issues," Dr. Lutfi would argue. They are "religious and moral [practices] that have been occurring in a legal vacuum" (*al-Ahram* 12.10.1995).[5] For him and many others, the patients called "brain dead" are actually "beating-heart-bodies (*al-Ahram* 16.12.1995; *al-Akhbar* 14.6.1997). Specializing in the technical aspects of brain death, he reports that in 70 percent of the cases labeled as brain dead, part of the brain cells [part of the brain *or* some of the brain cells] continue to work, the growth hormone continues to be secreted, and a number of voluntary movements can be detected. Furthermore, some involuntary reactions such as bleeding occur in the case of incision (*al-Wafd* 22.3.1997). Life here is seen as a function of growth, which results from conscious as well as unconscious forces.

This debate is a cultural site for the social production of authoritative knowledge and cultural facts to represent life and death within the existing social relations of power. As Kaufman and Morgan note, corpses could be cold and silent, but they are given words and meanings, spoken, embraced, staved off, and otherwise patterned (Kaufman and Morgan 2005: 319). I assume such diversity stems from social relations of power intricately connected to processes of establishing the value of the body within more general processes of social production. This idea receives impetus because the organs discourse is saturated with intense sense of distrust not about the dead body *per se*, but around issues of injustice and inequality taking place under a corrupt state and relations of production marked by an exacerbated sense of bias for those who have money but are not necessarily committed to moral principles represented by a tradition that is allegedly shared by all.

The anti-brain death proponents view it as a sign of losing "the sanctity of all human rights, including those of the dead" (*al-Sha'b* 6.4.1997). Such ideas would also appeal to other collective sentiments and morals presenting Egypt as an integrated body threatened by brain death related practices perceived as involving some unfair exchange. Some interlocutors argue that the emergence of the concept of "brain death" was linked from the outset to an increased *market demand* for human organs. These interlocutors are mostly physicians. They deeply regret that most of the organs removed in conditions of "deep coma" belong to "second-rate citizens" or "African and Indian immigrants" whose lives are used to lengthen the lives of those who can pay the price demanded. They allude to issues of unequal exchange between the poor and the rich when they refuse that "bodies of Egyptians"—meaning those of the poor—be degraded to such a low position (*al-Ahram* 7.10.1995). These debaters argue on the grounds that the new technologies would serve the affluent part of society who would be enriched in illegal ways.

The media plays a double-edged role in all this. The views and news published are utilized by the interlocutors to argue against the whole idea of accepting organ transplantation as immoral. Many of the materials published are very hard to verify. However, verification in the case of rumors is beside the point. What matters is the effect such news can produce especially when some of their themes cannot be proved or annulled. In all cases, tinkering with the body in life and death is immoral and deserves extreme punishments. I argue that such penalties are demanded because the body is inseparable from life through the immortal notion of *al-nafs* as emblematic for a social omnipresent existential and transcendental commonality.

The media contributes to drawing a bleak image of the future using the issue of brain death. An example is caricature in the *al-Wafd* opposition newspaper (28.1.1996) showing three men dressed in prison uniforms each carrying a human organ while walking out of a place carrying the sign, "The University Hospital Butcher," and "Wholesale and Trial." The image carries symbols representing major aspects of society including the government, the health system, education, and law. All are viewed as corrupt and collectively represented by the symbolic value of the body.

Different opinions on the issue of brain death should be interpreted as statements of truth that somehow express the interests of those who promote them and those who resist making them freely available. In other words, I view these debates as one field of power struggle indirectly addressing the immoral issue of using the bodies of some for the empowerment of others

(Comaroff and Comaroff 1999: 282). These debates certainly occur against a background of horror; the media is saturated with stories of organ theft carried out by surgeons and ordinary people alike (*al-Ahram* 7.10.1995).[6] Whether these stories are true or not is secondary to my argument. They are very widely circulated in newspapers, TV shows, radio talks, cyber networks, and so forth.

In a comparable situation in South Africa, Comaroff and Comaroff venture into linking local realities to abstract analytical categories including colonization, globalization, and postcolonialism in South Africa. Their ethnographic context is focused on issues of magic and witchcraft. In brief, the context is composed of an occult economy where young adults assault and burn elderly people believed to have seized their wealth in immoral ways. The case in Egypt is of course different. However, I hold that the same political economic forces working at the global level ultimately shape it. According to the authors in that context "witches distil complex material and social processes into comprehensible human motives, then they tend to figure in narratives that tie trans-local processes to local events, that map trans-local scenes onto local landscapes, that translate trans-local discourses into local vocabularies of cause and effect" (Ibid: 286). I would suggest that a comparable operation is taking place in Egypt with regard to the notion of *al-nafs*. On one hand, the market presents production and reproduction operations that could defy comprehension by ordinary people. The observation that a few men became extraordinarily rich and in no time is a riddle that defies ordinary ways of explanation. Egyptian men and women often tend to resort to associating these observations with the power of God. When it is noticed that someone has become rich in a noticeably short period of time they would say *rabbina fatah 'alaih wi 'alluh khud* (God has opened paths to wealth for him). In all cases it seems that neoliberal economics have pervaded society to the extent that the phenomenon of rapid enrichment became a dream of many people belonging to different classes.

Some who would reject such rapid enrichment because it is possibly associated with criminal acts would demand that extreme penalties be applied to those proven guilty. The case of body and body theft is a perfect example. Firstly, they would highlight that the body is also a divine mystery inaccessible to ordinary people. The notion of *al-nafs* is readily available. It is the sacred property of God. Those who violate its sanctity commit an unforgivable transgression and should be severely punished. Most prominent among the nationalist interlocutors is the columnist Waghih Abu Zikra of al-Akhbar paper, who warns, "if the trade in organs is officially instituted, a few 'deviant physicians' would massacre the rest of the Egyptian body" (*al-Ahrām* 23.5.1997). On a different occasion this overtly nationalist rhetoric turns into a defense of the lower classes, or "the poor." The columnist celebrates a decision by Parliament which rejects organ transplantation: "The decision will prevent the process of selling human organs for very high prices that only the fortunate classes in Egypt and other Arab countries could afford" (*al-Akhbar* 30.5.1997). Implied here is a class conflict on two scales. One is within Egypt where it would threaten the social order because it would allow the rich to further exploit the poor and thus jeopardize social cohesion. The other is global; the Egyptians as a whole represent a nation that is materially poorer than the neighboring oil-rich countries, and the inhabitants of such oil-rich sheikhdoms.

Al-nafs that the anti-brain death debaters conjure up feels pain. A scholar from al-Azhar takes this thought further. Imam Jad el-Haq Ali, who also was the Grand Imam of al-Azhar before Imam Tantaawy, argues that the dead body remains sensitive to the outside world and feels pain. The Imam backs his thought by one Hadith which reports the Prophet as saying, "breaking the bones of the dead is similar to breaking those of the living" (*al-Wafd* 28.1.1996).[7] It is a general belief anyway that dead bodies are ultimately connected to exact particular *nufūs*. These are believed to remain alive after the bodies perish. There, they *feel* pleasure and pain toward events in the world of their descendants, especially those related to acts performed by their descendants. In other words, they continue to be present in the social world and contribute to shaping people's feelings and actions. Examples to illustrate this point are numerous in Egyptian social life. Most prominent is when people read the Quran or give offerings to the poor or visit Mecca on pilgrimage. At times they carry out these deeds on behalf of their deceased relatives who they believe are in touch with them forever and are pleased by their blessed deeds. *Al-nafs* of the relative is imagined to be pleased by these acts of piety. It would be angry and unhappy by sinful acts. Egypt is a unique example among other Muslim countries as it is where the dead are buried in family graveyards on top of the ground in small rooms that are continually visited. Interestingly, these practices are viewed by Dr. Hamdy al-Sayyed as obstacles to accepting the notion of brain death.[8]

In contrast, medical care offers a sharp line separating the living body from the dead body. The former can be a person. The latter is not. The law, however, does not maintain this separation. A dead body belongs to a deceased person with rights operating after their departure. Furthermore, in Islamic tradition persons pass through death to become spirits who are reconstructed and reintegrated into social relations as ancestors (cf. Kaufman and Morgan 2005). Additionally, biomedicine presents life as something associated with health and well-being. Death, in contrast, is associated with nothingness. Simultaneously, the biomedical concept of brain death suggests that the incapacitated "dead" thing can still assist life because its parts can be integrated into other bodies. So biomedicine itself contributes to the liminality of the body it calls brain dead.

Al-nafs in Islamic imaginations is somewhat *liminal*; it continues to exist in the minds of the living as a disembodied state of being waiting to reunite with the body on the day of resurrection. This same force is the subject of intense speculation in brain death that throws light on some of its important meanings in current society. Critics of brain death use the example of pregnancy to argue that life is a continuous line connecting between different bodies. The example consists of pregnant women regarded as brain dead but who continued to show several signs of life, such as their ability to support a continuous blood flow for the whole body which helps these bodies to grow, and, most significantly, to give birth. These ideas connect to the religious concepts of the spirit or *al-nafs*, which never vanishes after death. For another physician, life consists of the ability of the body to maintain or reproduce life. This view is based on an example, repeatedly mentioned in the press, of women diagnosed as "brain dead" while being pregnant. Their pregnancy was maintained for five months in some cases (*al-Ahram* 11.6.1996), and until the moment of giving birth to "*healthy* children" (*al-Ahram* 12.10.1995). Life here is seen as a continuous line connecting the mother with her living fetus. This latter perception reveals that life is not a property of the individual-self.

Crucial to the notion of brain death is the fact that the bodies labeled as such could confer life to other bodies through granting "material" organs that are attached to symbolic, emotional, and, thus, exchange values. This means the concepts must ultimately refer to relations of production generally perceived as set in favor of the more powerful. Tradition at this juncture is differentially interpreted to correspond to conflicting positions. The divisions within the discourse on brain death find explanation in the debate over donation of organs by the living from material rewards.

ORGAN DONATION

An issue that illustrates the disagreements on brain death is the one about giving body parts for material rewards. It often leads to the question of "who owns the body." The Grand Imam of al-Azhar sought by the pro-donation debaters responds that "God owns the whole universe . . . He put the body at our disposal to handle it in legitimate ways" (*al-Ahram* 31.1.1997). Nevertheless, who decides on the legitimacy of the processes of organ transplantation and their good or bad consequences on the suppliers and the recipients? Ultimately, the Imam's argument would lead to giving authority to his allied pro-donation medical professionals to decide on these matters, as he argues somewhere else (*al-Wafd* 22.3.1997). No definite answers to this question are offered, a fact that gives ground for those opposed to the new technologies to offer alternative answers conveyed within different moral sensibilities that are linked to opposing political strategies.

Fatwas in general, unlike the way they are presented to the public, are nonbinding opinions or advice. They are produced through highly speculative interpretations of complex texts composed of polysemic terms and metaphorical expressions. Some of the *fatwas* themselves become subject to interpretation by different segments of the public, especially those with opposing political and material interests. The *fatwa* mentioned above is not an exception. In general, however, one could say that a large part of the official religious institution has taken the side of the mainstream medical establishment and the state to support the new technologies. In the best cases, they gave the physicians, or what they call "*Aṣḥāb al-'ikhtiṣāṣ*," full authority to decide on these issues. They would generally remind all those concerned of the major principles of being honest, faithful, and fearful of God.

The only important exception is Sheikh Muhammad Mitawalli al-Sha'raawi, who is viewed by the public as an independent scholar in these debates. In the words of one Member of Parliament, the sheikh "has his freedom," while others, such as the Grand Imam and the Mufti, do not. The latter are ultimately "government Muftis," according to a Member of Parliament writing for the weekly *al-Dustour* (27.11.1996). Al-Sha'raawi is an example of a religious and political figure known for his ability to make scholarly ideas and views accessible to the general "public." Furthermore, he has taken the unique position of provisionally accepting organ transplantation. He argues that the human body was a gift from God and should not be tampered with. His idea is that "donating human organs was tantamount to opposing God's will by seeking to make a human being live longer than he or she is destined to" (*al-Ahram Weekly* 25.6.1998). Organ transplantation is thus *ḥarām* (impermissible or prohibited) because humans do not own their bodies: "They don't own the whole, so how could they own the parts?" the sheikh asks (*al-Akhbar* 5.6.1997). Nevertheless, the sheikh's position changed when he judged the following specific case. A man with renal failure was advised to receive a kidney transplant. His brother offered to donate a compatible kidney. The man carried health insurance through his employer, which specified that he should receive the therapy at a particular hospital. The surgeon in charge refused to perform the operation unless the patient brought a *fatwa* from Al-Sha'raawi stating that the operation was permitted. When asked for that *fatwa* the sheikh said: "there is no problem if doctors decide that it is beneficial for the patient, given that the brother is willingly giving a kidney . . . God will reward the brother" (*al-Ahram* 16.12.1995). This incident then underscores the significance of case-based law in Islam and the centrality of family relations as opposed to market-based transactions in deciding over the body and life.

The above view is taken by physicians who have learned the Quran and the *Hadith* and thus developed independent opinions about how certain medical questions should be viewed from an Islamic point of view. Most of the arguments raised by these physicians are focused on the question of "who owns the body" in life and after death. A physician concerned with showing published an example in al-Akhbar that many Quranic verses "clearly prohibit the donation of organs" (*al-Akhbar* 14.5.1997). For the physician God exclusively owns the body. The thoughts of the physicians link with the position of al-Sha'raawi, mentioned above (*al-Akhbar* 5.6.1997). An opposition paper, *al-Sha'b,* also publishes other opinions by the Front of al-Azhar *'Ulama* leading to the same conclusion (*al-Akhbar*, 17.6.1997). The Quranic verses and the Hadiths that these people quote are very different from those quoted by the pro-transplant religious scholars. This observation lends support to the pluralistic nature of the discourse on the body and life.

Another example that substantiates people's suspicions is Dr. Mustafa Mahmood, a well-known physician, preacher, and benefactor of a major charitable society that includes a hospital offering affordable services to the poor. Dr. Mahmood is a highly trusted public figure. He has a great command over a great variety of knowledge that enables him to occupy a unique position in the popular interpretations of religion and technology and the relationship between science and technology. This major local authority over issues affecting the public also suspects that the central government is "plagued with disastrous problems" and thus incapable of performing morally serious operations as organ transplantations (*al-Akhbar* 9.5.1997).

The response of the anti-transplant debaters reveals an additional layer of the discourse. They would argue that the proclaimed donations should be prohibited because they occur in a defective moral order. Particularly, the vast distances separating the poor and the rich threaten social cohesion. Some would go further and argue that the transplants should not only be banned. They should also be pronounced prohibited (*ḥarām*) from a purely religious point of view. I would still argue that this position in Egypt is engendered by the widespread belief that organ transplantation is a process mainly driven by the search for profit, which is a sign of the increasing commodification of the body. Such processes, many would argue, will eventually lead to the disintegration of the national body because it will deepen the divisions between its different constituents. In reaction, all the interlocutors ask for a ban on organ transplantation. Many of them argue that the body is ultimately owned by God and not by the persons who live by it.

It is hard to observe and meet with people who donated organs in Cairo and even harder to meet those who received body parts. The one I met was a middle-class woman who could afford to pay compensation for a kidney donor for her deceased husband who died shortly after the operation. The woman was open enough to narrate the story, although only in broad outline. She is a high-ranking bureaucrat in a public university. Her husband was a professor in the same place. They both inherited land from their original families that enabled them to lead a comfortable life. The husband suffered kidney failure after a long struggle with disease. The "donor" was paid a sum of money that he used to buy a microbus to operate a taxi service. The income enabled him to improve his family's living conditions, according to the recipient's wife. Shortly, however, "he died in a horrible accident in his new car; the new job might have been too hard for him, especially after losing one kidney," the lady suspects with an obvious sense of regret. "Also, the transplanted kidney was rejected," she goes on with a sense of blaming the doctors who were too enthusiastic about performing the operation. The family could afford another transplant. The doctors were ready to perform it too. However, the patient chose not to have it although he was sure he was going to die shortly after that decision. The widowed woman was obviously very sad. Not only about her husband; also about the man who "donated," or rather sold, his kidney. She thought it was a horrible thing to take someone else's body part in return for money. The attitude of this person must be common among many people, especially given the centrality of the belief that health is not something that can be bought for money. It is a far more complex notion characterizing social harmony that springs from a sustainable sense of morality and correctness. The sense of blame and regret links well with the notion of *al-nafs al-lawwāmah* described earlier. Particularly, the body issue is perceived indirectly through a substantial layer of moral discourse resisting reduction of the body to a commodity.

Organ transference rarely involves a process of donation based on altruism. There is ample evidence that it occurs between people occupying very different positions and endowed with disparate privileges. In brief, the flow of organs goes from the poor to the rich who provide monetary compensation. This practice ultimately relates to the larger issue of the cultural meanings of the gift and the problem of social redistribution (Titmuss 1970: 71–89). In a context where the categories of social class play a major role in the way people judge different opinions and decisions, and where a corrupt state has given way to the development of a free-market economy, the physicians' call and approval of the Imam is viewed by the public as inevitably associated with the despised trade in living organs. It is common knowledge in

Cairo that selling organs would always involve "poor" suppliers and "rich" recipients.[9] It is automatic that the calls above are met with a great amount of suspicion and rejection. They are interpreted in contexts of relationships between the rich and the poor, the ruler and the ruled, the powerful and the dispossessed. All these have been characterized by a strong sense of distrust and unfairness. This latter thought gives ground for the opponents of organ transplantation to reject these practices because they link to profound issues of social injustice characterizing the social structure and distribution of economic wealth in society as a whole.

CONCLUSION

We learn from the above debates that personhood does not reside in the physical or cognitive existence of the individuals concerned. It is a collective property. Second, persons are produced in a tradition and discourses that are essentially social. Third, knowledge used in the debates is an index for the power relations that determine who lives and who dies.

In the Egyptian context the notion of *al-nafs* plays a major role in shaping people's perceptions and feelings about the body. The debates above help identify further attributes of this category. First, it identifies with the idea of growth and ability to give birth that in turn refers to issues of social reproduction. The incapacitated body that is termed as brain dead is interpreted by the opponents as having been or being a *nafs* that is able to enliven another, make it grow, and even produce some labor that would lead to reproduction. In their understanding, therefore, the bodies called "brain dead" by the hegemonic discourse are kept within the plural system of knowledge that views life as a continuous line characterizing *al-nafs* that cuts across death as conventionally defined. Second, it emphasizes the forms of life manifest in the heart-beating bodies as elements of power because they are able to grow and reproduce.

Second, it is a property of persons rather than physical bodies. It exists in *al-nafs* that operates in this and the other world. Likewise, health and sickness are properties of mindful rather than mere physical bodies. They also form a continuum and are not separate categories, as discussed in previous chapters.

Third, it is a religious concept, which is a fact that makes much of the discourse on it sound like a moral theology with a normal space for *al-Sharī'ah*. Ebrahim Moosa notes that textbooks, legal opinions, and scholarly discourses of the Islamic tradition "indicate that the law responded to very real life conditions and addressed the needs of the societies it served. Legal theory, as a meta-theory, reflected the contemporary sociopolitical realities. In other words, even a law colored by overt religious imperatives has a functional sociology and anthropology" (1999: 307). Wael Hallaq (1999) also stresses that the judges who have worked in this field have been produced by their own communities as legal experts qualified to fulfill a variety of functions that, in totality, made up the Islamic legal system. Furthermore, these experts knew about the social contexts of the individuals whom they served. Their knowledge formed a necessary condition for providing a service suited at the same time to local traditions and divine justice. The professional map for those who worked in this field must have been very complex given the variety of expertise available. For the present context however it suffices to know that the persons who provided legal services based on *al-Shari'ah* for the public were known as *muftiyīn*, author-jurists, judges, and law professors (Barber 2007: 8–13).

The debates above indicate that all would claim that their final goal is the "common good" of society. The pro-donation debaters translate mainstream biomedical arguments. Nevertheless, I would conclude that despite their straightforwardness, there is what Strathern (1992) calls a "domaining effect," which has to do with the cultural life of ideas, "in those habits of thought about which for most of the time we are very much unaware, the ideas that reproduce themselves in our communications *never reproduce themselves exactly*" (Strathern 1992: 6, emphasis original). More profoundly, upon their reproduction in different contexts ideas are stamped by the modes social life has produced and reproduced in the societies concerned. The terms used in this stamp are determined by these societies' tradition. Therefore, the resulting discourse, including the reaction against organ donations, thus forms an index for the local society including dominant power relations.

NOTES

1. One such film appeared as early as 1989 and starred major actor Noor al-Sherif who plays the role of a taxi driver named Qurashi who runs to help a man who suffers a car accident by taking to him to hospital. The victim happens to be a wealthy businessman who owns a hospital. Doctors require a blood transfusion, and Qurashi happens to be of a compatible blood group. He donates his blood and refuses to take compensation of any kind. The rich man, impressed by the high morals of the poorer fellow, offers him a job as his private chauffeur. Qurashi is then well treated, housed, and fed at the home of his grateful benefactor, who still needs further treatment. The employer owns a share in a private hospital. One of his partners is a physician who manages to make Qurashi believe he needs an operation for some pain that the physician has artificially induced. Long after the operation, Qurashi discovers that his kidney was "stolen" in this operation. With help from a lawyer and a physician, Qurashi manages to sue the businessman and the physician. In court he demands that his

kidney be returned to his body. The court decides that although the kidney removal has been proven, there is no legal precedent to support the victim's demand or to prosecute those who removed the body part. In a dramatic final scene that shifts between Qurashi, the judge, the lawyers, and a portrait of President Mubarak, Qurashi addresses the president: "Are you content with this? We are robbed down to our flesh."

2. See for example Lutfi (1992).

3. For a global report, see Scheper-Hughes 2000. Case studies describing specific contexts include Sharp 2000 on the United States, Papagaroufali 1999 on Greece, and Lock 1996 on Japan.

4. This opinion of the Imans was announced in a conference organized by the Assembly of Islamic Research Affiliated with al-Azhar.

5. It is not true that these debates occur in a legal vacuum, as many of the debaters argue. The press indicates, however, that the current legal codes are not able to deal with the complexity of the issues under discussion. Dr. Ahmad Sa'd, professor of civil law in Cairo University, reports that the current legal codes are too old and thus inappropriate to deal with ethical questions posed by the recently emerging technologies of life. The only law about the dead body, for example, was issued in 1937. The professor quotes Material No. 160, paragraph 3, of the penal law issued by Law 58 in 1937, which places a penalty of less than a year in prison, or a charge of no more than fifty pounds, on everyone who has violated the sanctity of, or desecrated, tombs. The professor continues: "The legislator has convicted everyone who violates the sanctity of the tombs or graveyards, or desecrates them [. . .] meanwhile; however, the legislator unfortunately considered the body as owned by no one. If someone removes an organ from the dead body, the legislator would not consider that removal as a criminal act, but a violation (*intihaak*). Whereas if there are assets buried with the dead and someone takes them, the law views this act as a crime. This is a shortcoming in Egyptian legislation" (*al-Wafd* 26.1.1996). As a result, however, the existing laws are inappropriate to deal with the issues in question (*al-Wafd* 26.1.1996; see also *al-Ahram* 12.10.1995).

6. The stories or rumors on this issue are countless. For older examples, see *al-Akhbar* 9.5.1997 and *al-Ahram* 11.6.1996. The World Wide Web provides innumerable narratives that supposedly occur in Egypt but are well connected to the regional and world scenery of illicit economies profiting from human organs. For a current example see www.youm7.com/News.asp?NewsID=454390.

7. The same Hadith and thoughts were also published in *al-Wafd* on 26.1.1996 and 23.3.1997.

8. This particular note is published in the website of Dr. Mohammad al-Qaradawi who is also a great enthusiast for organ transplantation (www.qaradawi.net/2010-02-01-08-43-29/4600.html) on 11 March 2009.

9. I prefer using the term "suppliers" rather that the term "donors." The latter term implies a sense of voluntarism that is hardly available in contexts such as giving blood or organs as Titmuss's (1970) study so sharply demonstrates in the context of blood "donation" (*ibid*: 238).

5

Ethnography as Social Critique

This book has dealt with one particular section of social life in Cairo: It focuses on how individuals and families experience living conditions subjectively. In this chapter I conceptualize the whole study in terms of *al-nafs* in connection with anthropological analytical concepts of local biology and subjectivity. I think *al-nafs* is an "idiomatic" expression useful for understanding local traditions in their own terms. It offers an opportunity to conduct ethnography as cultural critique, because it shows how life conditions are subjectively reworked, articulated, debated, and contested by different actors. It is a discursive practice helpful to appreciate the complexity of social life as it aligns itself with practical reason that benefits from its subjective, uncertain, flexible, adapting, and empowering aspects to run everyday struggles for coping with and accommodating increasingly uncompromising social and economic conditions of modern life. I should however note that *al-nafs* is by no means a static and unchanging notion in isolation from other similar concepts. On the contrary, it is a traditional notion embedded within contemporary discourses of power.

The aspects of *al-nafs* are explored in four main spaces. The first includes health practitioners who utilize *al-nafs* to conceptualize life as an integrated totality. Only one of the manuals that I discussed in this study attempted to reconcile the notion of *al-nafs* with perspectives of modern psychiatry. All the other manuals are construable as a response to crises experienced by modern society and excessively materialist biomedicine. The second aspect of *al-nafs* focuses on its capacity to mediate between individual and society through the family. The third aspect of *al-nafs* focuses on emotions and their utility to explain ill health not in pure physical terms but rather critical holistic terms. The capacity of *al-nafs* to conduct social critique is evident in this case; a biomedical category focused on physical causes of ill health is remade into an avenue for moral critique. The fourth aspect further focuses on the moral, religious, and eschatological dimensions of *al-nafs,* which operate as means of empowerment as they assist people to engage their society's moral concerns in committed and nevertheless autonomous modes of reflection and action. The rest of this chapter includes notes on additional aspects of *al-nafs* and how they respond to the ethnographic descriptions in the former parts of the study. Finally, I discuss further aspects of *al-nafs* using the notion of discursive tradition.

Cartesian sciences generally assume that the body is readily accessible to the materialist gaze of empiricist knowledge and controllable by "physical" and "psychological" means used jointly or separately. This general approach and its techniques have long been revisited and reconsidered. No need here to make a straw man out of them. One example however may be necessary to show that the critique of this perspective came out from within those who once celebrated it; that is, the edited volume by Kleinman, Brodwin, *Good and Good* (1994) focuses on pain as human experience. The introductory chapter of that book confirms the dissatisfaction of the authors with the existing approaches to human life and well-being. They report that even the field called "psychosomatic medicine" that has been striving to overcome shortcomings resulting from the well-known separation of the body and mind has been one of the least developed areas of studies and research.

I agree with this. But what I am trying to say is something slightly different. I think the problem is not simply the construction of the mind and body as if they were separate or where one is active and the other is passive. The issue is that this whole separation and the attempts to overcome it have been taking place within modern biomedicine which belongs to western societies. These should not remain unexamined especially in a comparative discipline like anthropology. Comparison presumes distance from the subjects included which is supposed to free ethnographic studies and other kinds of research from long-lasting forms of centrism.

The body is *lived* and *experienced* by individuals whose ways of sensing, feeling, and thinking about the world are diversely shaped *within* families and communities who also act as groups to live and prosper in diverse and changing circumstances. And the body is inseparable from those long-standing authoritative traditions reproduced by and within these communities. My argument is: within these traditions the idea of the body has been evolving in ever unique ways. The specific minutiae and trajectories of those traditions must have shaped the meanings of the body as well as its physiology. My general suggestion in this book has been to shift the attention away from both the presumably objective physical realities as well as the subjective experiences. We should focus on *life* as represented by *al-nafs* as a culture-specific space for shaping and reshaping the body and mind and the complex ways they are experienced. It is crucial to emphasize in this context that the body is constructed in compounded ways including the views of the study's respondents as well as the experiences of the observer.

Al-nafs is a relational concept representing the subjects included in the study. It mediates dyadic and collective interactions of social groups as mutually dependent wholes. Most fascinating about it is that it responds to the scholarly notion of "local biology" and "mindful bodies" discussed above. It brings together the material and the immaterial, the thinkable and the unthinkable, the real and the unreal, the visible and the imagined, as well as the sensed and the felt into one unit which is *life*. In addition, it presents a form of complex cultural critique; it takes issue with the Cartesian body/mind duality while keeping a distance from the Durkheimian collective consciousness as well as the Freudian super ego. The meaning of *al-nafs* is very similar to the anthropological notion the subject as discussed in the introductory chapter.

A far more interesting dimension of *al-nafs* appears when it is viewed as a "discursive tradition"—a concept reproduced via continual rethinking of the founding texts of the Islamic tradition in connection to everyday life concerns. My ethnographic descriptions and interpretations of life in Cairo agree, though in uneven ways, with the results of Moosa's (2005) textual analyses of the notion of *al-nafs* in the writings of Abu Hamid al-Aghazali. This is a very well-known scholar and mystic who lived between 1058 and 1111 AD. He studied, taught, and authored many books most significantly in Damascus, Jerusalem, Mecca, Medina, and Baghdad. His influence is still evident in the contemporary Muslim world including of course Cairo. His multi-volume *Resuscitation of the Sciences of Religion* is now circulated probably more than ever before; it has been endlessly reprinted and lately posted on the Web for free worldwide access along with other scholarly works expounding and commenting on it.

The reason Moosa's work is interesting is multifold. First, al-Ghazali actually presumed a kind of *imagination* rather than formal knowledge. It is fascinating to think of the way "mystical practices" of Islam spread to different extents in different parts of society. On the way it contributed to schooling the self and conscience of individuals and groups. These acquire this kind of education through their integral parts of wider social as well as cosmic realities. These realities were assumed to exist in a state of harmony and symmetry that humans had to learn, sustain and develop. Most crucial among the kinds of knowledge that humans learn is *self-knowledge*, which operates to regulate behavior through *al-nafs*, which under certain conditions can turn the self into a "blaming or lamenting self, a self that enjoins vice, or a contented self" (Moosa 2005: 229).

Second, the knowledge of *al-nafs* is *intimate*. It enhances one's admiration for, reverence of, and confidence in God as the highest sovereign. Interestingly there is a condition for this knowledge to be distinctive from a mere factual accounting of the universe. To be so it has to start with the human *self*, which is a function of *al-nafs*. It should enable the subjects involved to stand in awe of God, the initial and ultimate sustainer. Moosa is right to suggest that such knowledge is represented by the notion of *adab*. This notion covers a wide range of virtues including politeness, good or high social taste, being creative and imaginative as well as respectful. *Adab* is instilled in individuals as public actors (Moosa 2005: 220). This is comparable to Mauss's (1970 [1935]) notion of habitus which was later adopted by Bourdieu (1998 and 1995) and many others. In social science terms of course this notion assists in interpreting *al-nafs* as a social capacity working toward minute "attuning" of human subjects in accordance with the prevailing tradition.

Third, most interesting to my research is the way the notion of *al-nafs* is constructed as a *dialogical relationship* between the macro and micro politics, namely, between the governance of the polis and the governance of the body. The human body and intellect, the spirit and whole existence are ultimately expressions of one sovereign power, which is God. *Al-nafs* in this sense is relational and mediating. Therefore it must be flexible, adaptive, uncertain, resistant, and obedient all at once. This is *al-nafs* as *polyvocal*. It has to engage a complex, diverse, and inexact terrain of thoughts, emotions, feelings, and virtues collectively constituting social life. *Al-nafs* therefore has to be critical of the very idea of bounded constructions. One solution for al-Ghazali and many others is to use metaphorical language. Metaphors and tropes therefore stand for "aesthetic sensibility that one experiences as subject: "it is the aesthetic dimension of any kind of subjectivity, irrespective of whether that subjectivity is in search of the divine or is the subject of artistic, ethical, or musical discourse" (Moosa 2005: 234). Accordingly, the *'aql* or intellect relates to the body like a king or ruler to his kingdom or city-state. But the ultimate essence of humans is not the intellect. It is the *heart* which in al-Ghazali's view is a faculty for perception, knowledge, and experience. al-Ghazali describes *al-nafs* (soul) in terms interchangeable with those used to describe the heart—"the subtle entity" that is the self of human beings, or their essence and identity (cf. Moosa 2005: 226).

Al-Ghazali conceptualizes this notion in metaphysical terms tightly linked and explained in contexts of a society experiencing endemic forms of corruption comparable to the one striking today's Cairo. The desire for ethical rectitude, Moosa notes, was the central challenge of that time which made self-knowledge indispensable as well as inescapable. Of course this kind of knowledge cannot be expected to be spread evenly among different persons and social groups.

Before proceeding I should make some precautionary notes. It is true that the classical notion of *al-nafs* could describe much of the current practices to maintain life and alleviate pain. This very concept is simultaneously embedded in an entirely contemporary modern society provided with a plural health system. The latter includes a dominating medical system invested mainly in curative care. Second, a significant part of this system has invested in the very notion of *al-nafs* which must have influenced it as described in chapter 1. Third, *al-nafs* is surviving within a culture and society ruled by entirely new institutions including most significantly the nation-state and the commercial market. No doubt these institutions of power have influenced this notion as they brought it within a larger discourse on human life that is partly based on local tradition as well as incoming systems of thoughts and technologies as discussed in chapter 4. The product of this complex contemporary situation is neither the classical notion of *al-nafs* nor the incoming modern ones. It is not a hybridized form either as it has been fashionable to say lately. The current situation is characterized by an established nation-state and encroaching market system. My study shows that there are efforts to critically engage with the dominating discourses produced by these institutions. The results of these efforts have been uneven, I think. The common denominator between them is the fact that they make it necessary to *think for oneself* in order to devise new solutions for unprecedented problems and needs. Most necessary within this context is not to presume that this thinking must produce particular fruits or go in particular directions and not others. More interesting and relevant, I think, is to open ways for uncertainty and multiplication of cultural forms that may not be already in our imagination but inherent in the logic of the reason we employ to think and act on our everyday life. That is nothing less than practical reason.

The notion of *Ṣeḥḥah* described both in the introductory chapter and chapter 1 contributes to this practical reason-based perspective. First it requires serious attention to the notion of subject and subjectivity. *Al-nafs* is actually the *seat* for these two notions. Much of what has been offered by the practitioners in chapter 1 capitalizes on the notion of *al-nafs* in midst of a whole variety of other concepts rooted in different traditions. Further, all are employed in thinking about emerging problems and concerns of modern life. No doubt the production of the pamphlets have been a response to a growing market place hungry for new commodities for emerging needs and demands. *Al-nafs* in Arabic is the only translation for the psyche. We have seen how the Quranic meanings of this classical concept were merged and remade to fit current worldviews regarding the subject and subjectivity. Further, they have been utilized to conceptualize modern practical concerns of psychiatric care that are ultimately connected to issues of surveillance and panopticon. This conceptualization is not remote from the classical concept of *al-nafs*.

The pamphlets discussed are made for individuals' "self-help." They utilize the notion of *al-nafs* which certainly includes a regulatory mechanism implemented by and within tradition through the use of information and knowledge. These are employed in the governance of the social body through self-knowledge. Moosa confirms that al-Ghazali's construction of *al-nafs* in context of the universe is anthropomorphic. Humans seek power as earthly monarchs who strive for perfection. Constantly recurring signs of imperfection however cause them to compensate for the sense of incompleteness through the use of the "politics of presence."

My description of *Būlāq*, including its available medical resources, emphasizes the constant presence of the family in the life of individuals. This is of course a familiar theme in the ethnography of the Middle East and probably elsewhere. Notable in the present case however is the inclusion of passionate obligations as quintessential elements of the subjects' experiences of pain. Emotions in this context link directly to the notion of *al-nafs*. It brings in the issue of the *other* understood in terms of subjectivity and intersubjectivity. *Al-nafs* is a *relational* concept. The notion of *mu'āmalah* (transactions) lies at the heart of it. This is precisely the intersubjectivity of ethics or the constant feeling of having meaningful relations of responsibility toward others. From this angle, the notion of *al-nafs* refers to a completely integrated state of being reflecting well-being in both physical, spiritual, and moral terms. The latter is inherently social. As discussed earlier, individuals in this context should be described as *networked* or rather *reticulated* agents. As such, the notion of *al-nafs* simultaneously represents individuals and consciousness of their bodies as well as the social relations in which they live.

The same precaution mentioned above applies here. Families in *Būlāq* by no means offer a quintessential type for the rest of the city. Their life should not be viewed as representing a uniform type of cultural continuity either. Much of family life is juxtaposed by opportunities for individuals to live independently. Many of them would immediately choose to do that. But many cannot afford to do that. They are exposed to a variety of stimulations disseminated via the media to live separately as independent individuals. But even upon living separately, individuals in Cairo become subjects to multiple forms and ways for conceptualizing their new ways of life. These forms certainly include the views and habits instilled during upbringing saturated with collective forms of *al-nafs* tightly attached to their individual selves. Again, there is no easy way to represent how traditional views and ways of life are aligned in modern society. They don't exist separately. They are part and parcel of the larger field represented by the plural system discussed earlier.

The case of *'iḍḍaghṭ* well represents the state of having to live multiple obligations beyond the perceived capacity of the individual human being. To appreciate this social syndrome we have to reconsider and possibly abandon the once-fashionable distinction between disease and illness which is of course due to viewing the body as separate from the mind. We notice that the vast majority of the explanations for *'iḍḍaghṭ* ultimately lead to *malignant* emotions as some force operating within a host that failed to accommodate various forms of "*ḍughūṭ alḥayāh*." This last term literally means that pressures (*ḍughūṭ*) exert a sickening effect on *al-nafs*. Of course *al-nafs* survives and changes within a matrix that includes other notions rooted in modern psychiatry and other forms of practice. What should concern us here is the fact that this traditional notion continues to survive, adapt, and include new ways of thinking and explanation while preserving a sense of continuity rooted in tradition.

This sense is neither traditional nor modern. That separation would be a simplification. Because inherent in it is a practical reason that is not primarily concerned with this rather ideological distinction. Practical reason is critical by definition. An effect of this critique is a shift of focus off the body and mind, both at once. Instead, *al-nafs* is offered. But it works not to reproduce the field of psychosomatic medical care as several physician respondents suggest. It strives to bring in the *moral* dimension of well-being which is one of its major aspects. In a way *al-nafs* brings the psychological into the political and the political into the psychological as Mary-Jo et al. phrase it. An essential function of *al-nafs* is moral evaluation of the self (*al-dhāt*). The latter points to the individual self conceived within that of the "Other," which includes the sovereign divine and the community (cf. Moosa 2005 and Qutb 2005). *Al-nafs* in this sense transforms *'iḍḍaghṭ* into a means for launching a social critique based on moral evaluation of the human right to live well.

Living well means happiness (*sa'ādah*), which I could argue is one salient conclusion from all my observations and interviews in Cairo. Health does not mean absence of disease, physical fitness, mental integrity, or all these combined. Essential to the meaning of life in Cairo is a sense of being relaxed, tranquil, and at peace. *Sa'ādah* flourishes on harmony and integrity not merely in the body but in the social surrounding in the first place. It is the antonym of *ta'āsah* (misery) engendered by *nakad* (distemper) that may infest the highly appreciated sense of serenity or at least calm mood (*mizāg rāyi'*). This would agree with the notion of *al-nafs* examined in greater detail by Moosa (2005: 212). The search for this sense is not striving for perfection, which is a property for individuals who aspire to piety and moral rectitude. Others however would differ from those but only in degree. They would continue to view them and their practices as a standard to take moral and ethical decisions.

Al-nafs in this sense is a tradition-specific area of transference that mediates, represents, and critically engages with many other capacities that represent life conditions within specific social and economic circumstances characterizing today's Egypt. In a word it is an idiomatic term that is impossible to translate without feeling the life of those who use it. Of course representatives of biomedicine could do so when they use it as equivalent to the notion of the psyche for example. But they could do that only from positions that can be easily challenged when viewed in contexts of the local tradition.

One such critical ground is the collectivist dimension of *al-nafs* which relates to issues of the law, power, and justice. *Al-nafs* in this sense can be viewed as a field of *debatable power* circulating within larger spaces of subjectivity and intersubjectivity. Finally the issue of organ donation offers an opportunity to examine the notions of life, health, well-being, and death in context of the notion of *al-nafs* as a cognitive concept with legal and moral dimensions and implications about power and authority at the level of society at large.

In Muslim tradition *al-nafs* is a space for the subject and subjectivity to express idiosyncratic views and feelings and be simultaneously remade. Moosa is correct to suggest that subjectivity in that sense simultaneously encompasses and transcends the notion of the soul, self, or the person. In that sense individuals identify by "an inner self of their subjectivity." They could *think critically*. Then they may consider discrete aspects of the discursive formations within which they live but have become inappropriate to arbitrate their subjectivity. *Al-nafs* undertakes this role because it is a relational layer, a mediating transference between three more concepts: *al-'aql* (the intellect), *al-qalb* (the heart), and *al-rūḥ* (spirit). Accordingly, *al-nafs* constitutes a distinctive kind of psychology called *pectoral*; it refers to the area of the chest and breathing. Thus the term *al-nafs* shares root with the term *nafas* or breath. In this sense subjectivity may be viewed as a form of empowerment because it simultaneously grants a space to be subject to commands and another to willingly respond to it in fashions specific to the subjects involved (223–230). Compared to the objectivist views and ideas circulated by physicians and other debaters, therefore, the knowledge operated by *al-nafs* is *intimate*, *holistic*, *intersubjective*, and guided by abstract objective knowledge all at once. It stems from the subject's commitment, admiration, and trust in the sovereign divine "Other" and fellow human beings.

Interestingly, this notion of *al-nafs* is ultimately linked to *fiqh* or the law in ways distinctive to Muslim tradition. In chapter 4 I discussed Hallaq's

(1999) descriptions of the spectrum of permission and prohibition in *fiqh* that included a shade of five degrees including obligatory (*wājib or farḍ*), recommended (*mandūb or mustaḥabb*), indifferent (*mubāḥ*), disapproved of (*makrūh*), or forbidden (*ḥarām*). According to Moosa, all these legal categories address the heart that encompasses the imagination, the soul, the intellect, and the spirit, and of course the relational space of *al-nafs*. It is in this sense that the latter is actually a legal notion that qualifies the individuals involved to be accountable and responsible for their actions. Ideally, I would argue that it is this conceptualization that creates rooms for debating the ideas on organ donation. The individuals involved believe that as humans they are morally accountable for obeying God's command because they embody God's words on earth (*khulafā allaha 'ala al-'arḍ*).

This is the core of my idea that *al-nafs* is a form of empowerment and submission all at once. It provides moral grounds for discourses very critical of commercialization, commodification, and concomitant fragmentation of human relations associated with increased marketization of social life. It is true that most Muslims live by God-given rules. Nevertheless, the question of authority and who is authoritative and who is not remains open. This is very true in the field of ethics as we saw in the chapter on organ donation. Thus the dialogical continuum between individual and society is sustained to achieve the disciplining of the soul (*tahdhīb al-nafs*), the governance of the body (*siyāsat al-badan*), and the administration of justice (*ri'āyat*) in society (Moosa 2005). This latter issue is a recurrent theme in my own study especially in the case of organ donation. There, the ethical issues ultimately give way for people to contend health conditions as inherently political. At this juncture humans have to identify and represent a supposedly transcendent sovereign. Most powerful and empowering in the idea of *al-nafs* is the fact that it is defined along lines cutting across the body and mind, individual and society, life and death, and this world and the world of eternity.

Bibliography

Aamer, Galal. 2010. *Egypt is in Imp's Hand* (*Masr 'ala kaf 'Afrīt*). Cairo: Dar al-Ain Lilnashr.

Abd al-'Aziz, Mohammed Kamal. 1997. *kaifa tuhafith 'ala kilyatika wa tatajannab al-fashal al-kalawi* [How to Keep Healthy Kidneys and Avoid Kidney Failure]. Cairo: maktabit ibn sina.

———. 1992. *Sab' 'atibbaa' min al-tabi'a: al-'ilag bidun giraha aw ḍawḍā'* [Seven Doctors from Nature: Therapy with no Surgery or Drugs]. Cairo: dar altalaa'i'.

———. 1987. *'I'jaz al-quran fi hawassi al-insan: diraasah fi al-'anf wa al-'uthun wa al-hunjarah fi du' ai-tib wa 'ulum al-quran wa al-ḥadīth* [The Inimitability of the Quran in the Human Senses: A Study in the Nose, the Ear and the Pharynx in Light of the Quranic Sciences and the Prophet's Traditions]. Cairo: maktabat ibn sina.

Abd al-Hamid, Mohammed. 1934. *mushkilaat al-tibib fi missr*. n.p. Maktabat Saba'.

Abdalla, Ismail, and B. B. du Toit (eds.). 1985. *African Healing Strategies*. Aweri Trado Medical Books.

Abdallah, Mohammed Mahmoud. 1993. *al-tib fi al-quran wa al-snunna: beyna al-daa' wa al-dawaa'* [Medicine in the Quran and the Prophet's Traditions]. Cairo: maktabat zahran.

Abul-'Azayem, Gamal Madi. 1994. *Al-quran wa al-ṣiḥḥah an-nafsiyya: ta'ammulaat fi al-'aayat al-quraniyya al-muta'alliqa bi al-ṣiḥḥah al-nafsiyaa* [The Quran and the Psychological Health: Reflections on the Quranic Verses Relevant to the Psychological Health]. Cairo: dar al-hilal.

Abu-Lughod, Janet. 1971. *Cairo*: *1001 Years of the City Victorious*. Princeton, N.J.: Princeton University Press.

Abu-Lughod, Janet, and Ezz el-Din Attiya. 1963. *Cairo Fact Book*. Cairo: American University in Cairo, Social Research Centre.

Ad Hoc Committee of the Harvard Medical School to Examine the Definition of Death. 1968. "A Definition of Irreversible Coma." *Journal of the American Medical Association* 205(6): 337–40.

Al-Aswani, Alaa. 2010. *Why do the Egyptians not Revolt?* (*limātha lā yathūru al-misriyyūn*). Cairo: Dar al-Shorouq.
Al-Gamal, Ibrahim Mohammed. 1988. *Al-'istishfaa' bi al-Qruran* [Seeking Healing by the Quran]. Cairo: dar al-fadilah.
Al-Gamal, Ibrahim Mohammed Hassan. 1993. *'Amraad al-'asr bayna al-'ilm wa al-din* [The Disease of the Contemporary Times between Science and Religion]. Mansurah: maktabat al-'iman.
Al-Gammal, Samir Yahya. n.d. *Al-'ilaag al-shaafi bi al-nabataat al-tibbiyay* [Healing Therapies by Medicinal Plants]. Cairo: madbuli.
Al-Ghazali, Abu Hamid. 2008. *Iḥyā` 'Ulūm al-Dīne.* [Revival of Religious Sciences] Indonesia, Samaraqh: Kiryata Fotra Publishers.
Al-Hussaini, Ayman. 1990. *Humuum al-banaat* [The Girls' Concerns]. Cairo: maktabat ibn sina.
———. 1993a. *A'shaab wa nabataat fi khidmat al-jins al-latif* [Herbs and Plants in service of fair sex]. Cairo: maktabat ibn sina.
———. 1993b. *hal tu'uāni min 'irtifā' ḍaghṭ al-dam? Dawaa'uka min al-'a'shaab wa al-ghithaa'*. Cairo: Makatabat Ibn Sina.
———. 1993c. *Humuum al-mar'ah fi sin al-ya's* [Women's Concerns in the Menapause]. Cairo: dar al-talaai.
———. 1994a. *Wa daawini bi allati kaanat hiya al-daa'u: sayha gadida li al-tadaawi bi al-wasaa'il al-tabi'iyya* [Treat me by the Cause of my Illness: A New Call for Natural Therapies]. Cairo: maktabat ibn sina.
———. 1994b. *Al-sukkar wa l-ghitha' wa l-jins* [Diabetes, Nutrition, and Sex]. Cairo: dar al-talaa'i'.
Al-Kadi, Ahmed. 1995. "Contemporary Definition of Islamic Medicine." Paper presented at the Fifth International and First American Conference on Islamic Medicine, Orlando, Florida, April.
Al-Mahdi, Rabab, and Philip Marfleet. 2000. *Egypt: The Moment of Change*. London: Zed Books.
Al-Messiri, Nadim Nawal. 1977. "Family Relationships in a '*Hara*' in Cairo." In: Nicholas S. Hopkins and Saad Eddin Ibrahim (eds.), *Arab Society*, Pp. 212–222. Cairo: The American University in Cairo Press.
Al-Zabidi, Murtada. 1965. *Taj al-'Arus min Jawahir al-Qamus* [The Arabic Lexicon Taj al-Arus]. Kuwait: Government Press.
Amarasingham, Lorna Rhodes. 1980. "Movement among Healers in Sri Lanka: A Case Study of a Sinhalese Patient." *Culture, Medicine and Psychiatry* 4: 71–92.
Amin, Galal. 1988. *Whatever Happened to the Egyptians? Changes in Egyptian Society from 1950 to the Present*. Cairo: The American University in Cairo Press.
Amin, Samir. 1989. *Eurocentrism*. New York: Monthly Review Press.
Antes, Peter. 1989. "Medicine and the Living Tradition of Islam." In: Lawrence E. Sullivan (ed.), *Healing and Restoring Health in the World's Religious Traditions*, Pp. 173–202. New York: MacMillan.
Asad, Mohammed. 1980. *The Message of the Quran*. Gibraltar: Dar Al-Andalus.
Asad, Talal. 2003. *Formations of the Secular: Christianity, Islam, Modernity*. Stanford, Calif.: Stanford University Press.

———. 2000. "Agency and Pain: An Exploration." *Culture and Religion* 1(1): 29–60.

———. 1994. Ethnographic Representation: Statistics and Modern Power. *Social Research* Spring, 61(1): 55–88.

———. 1993. *Genealogies of Religion: Discipline and Reasons of Power in Christianity and Islam*. Baltimore and London: The Johns Hopkins University Press.

———. 1992. "Conscripts of Western Civilization." In: Christine Gailey, (ed.), *Dialectical Anthropology: Essays in Honor of Stanley Diamond*, Pp. 333–351. Gainesville: University Press of Florida.

———. 1986. "The Idea of an Anthropology of Islam." *Occasional Papers Series of The Centre for Contemporary Arab Studies*. Washington, D.C.: Georgetown University Press.

———. 1979. "Anthropology and the Analysis of Ideology." *Man* 14: 607–627.

Ashour, Zainab, et al. 1995. "The Egyptian National Hypertension Project (NHP): Design and Rationale." *Hypertension* 26(1) [part 1]: 880–85.

Austin, John Langshaw. 1962. *How to Do Things with Words: The William James Lectures Delivered at Harvard University* [edited by James O. Urmson]. Oxford: Clarendon.

Baer, H., Singer, M., and Johnsen, J. 1986. "Introduction: Toward a Critical Medical Anthropology." *Social Science and Medicine* 23(2): 95–98.

Banerji, D. 1985. "The Political Economy of Western Medicine in Third World Countries." In: J. McKinlay (ed.), *Issues in the Political Economy of Health Care*, Pp. 257–282. London: Tavistock.

———. 1981. "The Place of Indigenous and Western Systems of Medicine in the Health Services in India." *Social Science and Medicine* 15A: 109–114.

Benjamin, Walter. 1969. *Illuminations.* Translated by Harry Zoh. Edited and with an introduction by Hannah Arendt. Preface by Leon Wieseltier. New York: Schockenbooks.

Blumhagen, Dan. 1980. "Hyper-tension: A Folk Illness with a Medical Name." *Culture, Medicine and Psychiatry* 4: 197–227.

Bourdieu, Pierre. 1995. *Outline of a Theory of Practice*. Cambridge: Cambridge University Press.

———. 1998. *Practical Reason: On the Theory of Action.* California: Stanford University Press.

Brodwin, Paul. 1996. *Medicine and Morality in Haiti: The Context for Healing Power*. Cambridge: University of Cambridge Press.

Bürgel, J. Christoph. 1976. "Secular and Religious Features of Medieval Arabic Medicine." In Charles Leslie (ed.), *Asian Medical Systems: A Comparative Study,* Pp. 44–62. Berkeley: University of California Press.

Chatterjee, Prtha. 1995. *Texts of Power: Emerging Disciplines in Colonial Bengal*. Minneapolis, Minn.: University of Minnesota Press.

Clot Bey, Antoine B. 1840. *Aperçu Général Sur L'Egypte*. Paris: Fortin, Masson et Cie.

Coles Pasha, Charles. 1918. *Recollections and Reflections*. London: The Saint Catherine Press.

Colonna, Fann. 1999. "A Doctor by a Canal: A Presentation of a Person, from Nasser to Foucault." In: Sophy Day, Evthymios Papataxiarchis, and Michael Stewart (eds.), *Lilies of the Field: Marginal People who live for the Moment*, Pp. 212–236. Colorado: Westview Press.

Conerly, Casey and Robert B. Edgerton (eds.). 2005. *A Companion to Psychological Anthropology: Modernity and Psychocultural Change*. Oxford: Blackwell Publishing Ltd.

Comaroff, Jean. 1980. "Healing and the Cultural Order: The Case of the Barolong boo Ratshidi of Southern Africa." *American Ethnologist* 7(4): 637–77.

Csordas, Thomas J. 1994. "Introduction: The Body as Representation and Being-in-the-World." In: Thomas J. Csordas (ed.), *Embodiment and Experience: The Existential Ground of Culture and Self*, Pp. 1–24. Cambridge: Cambridge University Press.

———. 1993. "Somatic Modes of Attention." *Cultural Anthropology* 8(2): 135–156.

Csordas, Thomas J., and Arthur Kleinman. 1990. "The Therapeutic Process." In: Thomas M. Johnson and Carolyn F. Sargent (eds.), *Medical Anthropology: Contemporary Theory and Method*, Pp. 11–25. New York: Greenwood Press.

Cunningham, Alfred. 1912. *Today in Egypt*. London: Hurst & Blackett.

Das, Veena. 2000. "The Practice of Organ Transplants: Networks, Documents, Translations." In: Margaret Lock, Alan Young, and Alberto Cambrosio (eds.), *Living and Working with the New Medical Technologies: Intersections of Inquiry*, Pp. 263–287. Cambridge: University of Cambridge Press.

Davis, Susan Schaefer. 1988. "Convenience, Cost and Courtesy: Factors Influencing Health Care Choices in Rural Morocco." In: Christine I. Zeichner (ed.), *Modern and Traditional Health Care in Developing Societies: Conflict and Cooperation*, Pp. 59–73. New York: University Press of America.

Dewalt, Billie R., and Pertti J. Pelto (eds.) 1985. *Micro and Macro Levels of Analysis in Anthropology*. Boulder,Colo.: Westview Press.

Dressler, William. 1995. "Intracultural Diversity and the Sociocultural Correlates of Blood Pressure: A Jamaican Example." *Medical Anthropology Quarterly* 9(3): 291–313.

———. 1984. "Hypertension and Perceived Stress." *Ethos* 13(3): 265–283.

Early, Evelyn A. 1993. *Baladi Women of Cairo: Playing with an Egg and a Stone*. London: Lynne Rienner Publishers.

Early, Evelyn. 1988. "The *Baladi* Curative System of Cairo, Egypt." *Culture, Medicine and Psychiatry* 12: 65–83.

Egyptian Society for Hypertension. 1997. *The Egyptian Society for Hypertension: A Report on the Development, Goals, Activities, and Board of Directors*. The Society Records.

El-Gawadi, Muhammad M. 1987. *As-Sahha wal-tib fi misr* [Health and Medicine in Egypt]. Zagazig: Zagazig University Publications.

Elling, Ray. 1981. "Political Economy, Cultural Hegemony, and Mixes of Traditional and Modern Medicine." *Social Science and Medicine* 15A: 89–99.

———. 1981a. "The Capitalist World-System and International Health." *International Journal of Health Services* 11: 21–51.

———. 1981b. "Introduction: Relations between Traditional and Modern Medical Systems." *Social Science and Medicine* 15(A): 87–88.

El-Mehairy, Theresa. 1984. *Medical Doctors: A Study of Role Concept and Job Satisfaction: The Egyptian Case*. Leiden: E. J. Brill.

El-Sayyid, H., and Emad Al-din Nosseir (eds.). 1983. *Al-Tib Maridan* [When Medicine is Sick]. Cairo: Maktab al-nil li tabi‘ wa al-nashr.

Fahmi, Fuad Ali. n.d. *Al-'ilaag al-shamil bi kul al-wasa'il: al-turuq al-tabi'iyaa - al-taqlidiyaa, al-'a'shaab, al-'adwiya* [Comprehensive Ttreatment by all the Means Possible: The Natural Traditional Methods, the Herbs and the Therapies]. Cairo: No Publisher.

Farmer, Paul. 1988. "Bad Blood, Spoiled Milk: Bodily Fluids and Moral Barometers in Rural Haiti." *American Ethnologist* 15(1): 62–84.

Farquhar, Judith, and Margaret Lock. 2007. "Introduction." In: Judith Farquhar and Margaret Lock (eds.), *Beyond the Body Proper: Reading the Anthropology of Material Life*. Pp. 1–16. Durham: Duke University Press.

Fischer, Michael M. J. 1999. "Emergent Forms of Life: Anthropologies of Late or Postmodernities." *Annual Review of Anthropology* 28: 455–78.

Fischer, Michael, Byron Good, and Mary-Jo DelVecchio Good. 1988. "Emotions, Illness and Healing in Middle Eastern Societies." Special Issue of *Culture, Medicine and Psychiatry* 12(1): 1–7.

Foster, George. 1987. "World Health Organization Behavioral Science Research: Problems and Prospects." *Social Science and Medicine* 24(9): 709–717.

———. 1984. "Anthropological Research Perspectives on Health Problems in Developing Countries." *Social Science and Medicine* 18(10): 847–854.

Foster, George, and M. Anderson. 1978. *Medical Anthropology*. New York: Wiley.

Foucault, Michel. 1989. *The Birth of the Clinic: Archaeology of Medical Practice*. London: Routledge.

———. 1992. *The Archaeology of Knowledge*. London: Routledge.

Frank, Arthur W. 2001. "The Remission Society." In: Peter Conrad (ed.), *The Sociology of Health and Illness: Critical Perspectives*, 6th edition, Pp. 149–152. New York: Worth Publishers.

Frankenberg, Ronald. 1988. "Gramsci, Culture, and Medical Anthropology: Kundry and Parsifal? or Rat's Tail to Sea Serpent?" *Medical Anthropology Quarterly* 2: 324–337.

———. 1980. "Medical Anthropology and Development: A Theoretical Perspective." *Social Science and Medicine* 14B: 197–207.

Frankenberg, Ronald, and J. Leeson. 1976. "Disease, Illness, and Sickness: Social Aspects of the Choice of Healer in a Lusaka Suburb." In J. Loudon (ed.), *Social Anthropology and Medicine*, Pp. 223–58. New York: Academic.

———. 1973. "The Sociology of Health Dilemmas in the Post-Colonial World: Intermediate Technology and Medical Care in Zambia, Zaire and China." In: E. de Kadt and G. Williams (eds.), *Sociology and development*. London: Tavistock.

Gallagher, Nancy. 1990. *Egypt's Other Wars: Epidemics and the Politics of Public Health*. Syracuse, N.Y.: Syracuse University Press.

———. 1985. "What Happened to Islamic Medicine." In: B. M. du Toit and I. H. Abdalla (eds.), *African Healing Strategies*. Owerri: Trado Medics Books.

———. 1982. "Social Medicine and Middle East History." The Haworth Press, Inc.

Garro, Linda. 1988. "Explaining High Blood Pressure: Variation in Knowledge about Illness." *American Ethnologist* 15(1): 98–119.

Geertz, Clifford. 1968. *Islam Observed: Religious Development in Morocco and Indonesia*. Chicago: University of Chicago Press.

Gellner, Ernest. 1992. *Postmodernism, Reason and Religion*. London: Routledge.

———. 1993 [1981]. *Muslim Society*. Cambridge: Cambridge University Press.

Gilsenan, Michael. 1982. *Recognizing Islam: An Anthropologist's Introduction*. London: Croom and Helm.

———. 1973. *Saint and Sufi in Modern Egypt: An Essay in the Sociology of Religion*. Oxford: Clarendon Press.

Good, Byron, Michael Fischer, Sarah S. Willen, and Mary-Jo DelVecchio Good. 2010. *A Reader in Medical Anthropology: Theoretical Trajectories, Emerging Realities*. Oxford: Wiley-Blackwell.

Good, Byron. 1995. *Medicine, Rationality and Experience: An Anthropological Perspective*. Cambridge: Cambridge University Press.

———. 1977. "The Heart of What is the Matter: The Semantics of Illness in Iran." *Culture, Medicine and Psychiatry* 1: 25–58.

Good, Byron, and Arthur Kleinman. 1985. "Epilogue: Culture and Depression." In: Arthur Kleinman and B. Good (eds), *Culture and Depression: Studies in the Anthropology and Cross Cultural Psychiatry of Affect and Disorder*, Pp. 491–505. Berkeley: University of California Press.

Good, Byron, and Mary-Jo DelVecchio Good. 1992. "The Comparative Study of Greeco-Islamic Medicine: The Integration of Medical Knowledge into Local Symbolic Contexts." In: Alan Young and Charles Leslie (eds.), *Paths to Asian Medical Knowledge*, Pp. 257–271. Berkeley: University of California Press.

Good, Byron J., and Mary-Jo DelVecchio Good. 1982. "Toward a Meaning Centered Analysis of Popular Illness Categories: 'Fright Illness' and 'Heart Distress' in Iran." In: A. J. Marsella and G. M. White (eds.), *Cultural Conceptions of Mental Health and Therapy*, Pp. 141–166. Boston: D. Reidel.

Good, Byron J., and Mary-Jo DelVecchio Good. 1993. "Learning Medicine: The Construction of Medical Knowledge at Harvard Medical School." In: S. Lindenbaum and M. Lock (eds.), *Knowledge, Power and Practice: The Anthropology of Medicine and Everyday Life*, Pp. 81–107. Berkeley: University of California Press.

Good, Byron, Mary-Jo DelVecchio Good, and Robert Moradi. 1985. "The Interpretation of Dysphoric Affect and Depression in Iranian Culture." In: A. Kleinman and B. Good, (eds.), *Culture and Depression: Studies in the Anthropology and Cross Cultural Psychiatry of Affect and Disorder*, Pp. 369–428. Berkeley: University of California Press.

Good, Byron J., Mary-Jo DelVecchio Good, Sandra Teresa Hyde, and Sara Pinto. 2008. 'Postcolonial Disorders: Reflections on Subjectivity in the Contemporary World.' In: Mary-Jo DelVecchio Good, et al. (eds.) *Postcolonial Disorders: Ethnographic Reflections on Subjectivity*, Pp.1–40. Berkeley: University of California Press.

Good, Mary-Jo Delvecchio. 1995. "Cultural Studies of Biomedicine: An Agenda for Research." *Social Science and Medicine* 41(4): 461–473.

Good, Mary-Jo DelVecchio, Sandra Teresa Hyde, Sara Pinto, and Byron Good. 2008. "Postcolonial Disorders: Postcolonial Disorders: Reflections on Subjectivity in the Contemporary World." In Mary-Jo DelVecchio Good, Sandra Teresa Hyde, Sara Pinto and Byron Good (eds.), *Postcolonial Disorders*, Pp. 1–40. Berkeley: University of California Press.

Good, Mary-Jo DelVecchio, Paul E. Brodwin, Byron Good, and Arthur Kleinman. 1994. *Pain as Human Experience: An Anthropological Perspective*. Berkeley: University of California Press.

Gran, Peter, 1979a. "Medical Pluralism in Arab and Egyptian History: An Overview of Class Structures and Philosophies of the Main Phase." *Social Science and Medicine* 13(B): 339–48.

———. 1979b. *Islamic Roots of Capitalism: 1760–1840*. Austin: University of Texas Press for an history of Eighteenth century of Egypt illustrating development of capitalist relations of production well before the invasion of European powers.

Greenwood, B. 1981. "Cold or Spirits? Choice and Ambiguity in Morocco's Pluralistic Medical System." *Social Science and Medicine* 5B: 219–235.

Greenwood, Davydd, Shirley Lindenbaum, Margaret Lock, and Alan Young, 1988. "Introduction." *American Ethnologist* 15 (1): 1–3.

Gruenbaum, Ellen. 1981. "Medical Anthropology, Health Policy and the State: A Case Study of Sudan." *Policy Studies Review* 1(1): 47–65.

Hallaq, Wael. 1999. *A History of Islamic Legal Theories: An Introduction to Sunni Usul al-fiqh*. Cambridge: Cambridge University Press.

Hammady, Iman. 1990. *Religious Medical Centres in Cairo*. Unpublished M.A. Thesis. American University in Cairo.

Harraz, Abdul Rahman, and Yusuf Abul Hag. 1994. *Wasfaat shaikh al-'ashshabin 'Abdul Rahmaan al-Harraaz fi al-'ilaaj bi al'a'shaab* [Prescriptions of the Herbalists' Chief, Abdul Rahmaan al-Harraaz in Herb Therapy]. Cairo: Dar al-Lata'if.

Heggenhougen, Kris H. 2000. "More than just 'Interesting!': Anthropology, Health and Human Rights." *Social Science and Medicine* 50: 1171–1175.

———. 1987. "Traditional Medicine (in Developing Countries): Intrinsic Value and Relevance for Holistic Health Care." *Holistic Medicine* 2: 47–56.

———. 1980. "Bomohs, Doctors and Sinsehs: Medical Pluralism in Malaysia." *Social Science and Medicine* 14(B): 235–244.

Helman, Cecil. 1985. "Psyche, Soma, and Society: The Social Constitution of Psychosomatic Disorders." *Culture, Medicine and Psychiatry* 9: 1–26.

Hoodfar, Homa. 1997. *Between Marriage and the Market: Intimate Politics and Survival in Cairo*. Berkeley: University of California Press.

Ibrahim, Muhsin, et al. 1995. "Hypertension Prevalence, Awareness, Treatment, and Control in Egypt: Results from the Egyptian National Hypertension Project (NHP)." *Hypertension* 26(6) [part 1]: 886–890.

Inhorn, Marcia. 1996. *Quest for Conception: Gender, Infertility, and Egyptian Medical Traditions*. Philadelphia: University of Pennsylvania Press.

Janzen, John. 1985. "Changing Concepts of African Therapeutics: An Historical Perspective." In: B. M. du Toit and Ismael Abdall (eds.), *African Healing Strategies*, Pp. 61–81. Oweri Trado Medical Books.

———. 1978. *The Quest for Therapy in Lower Zaire*. Berkeley: University of California Press.

Khattab, Omar. 1985. *Aspects of the History of Imam Mahmoud Khattab Al-Sabki*. Cairo: Dar al-'I'tissaam. (In Arabic.).

Kleinman, Arthur. 1980. *Patients and Healers in the Context of Culture*. Berkeley: University of California Press.

Kleinman, Arthur; Leon Eisenberg and Byron Good. 1978. Culture, Illness and Care. Clinical Lessons fom Anthropologic and Cross-Cultural Research. *Annals of Internal medicine* 88: 251–258.

Kleinman, Arthur, Paul E. Brodwin, Byron J. Good, and Mary-Jo DelVecchio Good. 1994. Pain as Human Experience: An Introduction. In: Mary-Jo DelVecchio Good, Paul E. Brodwin, Byron J. Good, and Arthur Kleinman (eds.), *Pain as Human Experience: An Anthropological Experience*, Pp. 1–28. Berkeley: University of California Press.

Koselleck, R. 1988. *Critique and Crisis: Enlightenment and the Pathogenesis of Modern Society*. Cambridge, Mass.: MIT Press.

Kuhnke, Laverne. 1992. *Lives at Risk: Public Health in Nineteenth-Century Egypt*. Cairo: American University in Cairo Press.

Kuppinger, Petra. 1990. "El-Tayyibin: The Political Economy of a Cairene Low-Income Community." Unpublished M.A Thesis, The American University in Cairo.

Lane, Sandra, and Millar, Marcia. 1987. "The 'Hierarchy of Resort' Re-examined: Status and Class Differentials as Determinants of Therapy for Eye Disease in the Egyptian Delta." *Urban Anthropology* 16(2): 151–82.

Lazarus, Ellen, Merril Singer, and Hans Baer. 1990. "Critical Medical Anthropology." *Social Science and Medicine* 30(2): v–viii.

Leprette, Fernand. 1939. *Egypt: Land of the Nile*. Translated by Lillian Goar. Cairo: R. Schindler Printer and Publisher.

Leslie. 1980. "Medical Pluralism in World Perspective." *Social Science and Medicine* 14(B): 191–195.

Leslie, Charles (ed.). 1976. *Asian Medical Systems: A Comparative Study*. Berkeley and Los Angeles: University of California Press.

———. 1976a. "Pluralism and Integration in the Indian and Chinese Medical Systems. In: Arthur Kleinman, P. Kundstadter, E. R. Alexander, and J. L. Gale (eds.), *Medicine in Chinese Cultures*. DHEW Publication No. 75–653, National Institute of Health.

———. 1976b. "The Ambiguities of Medical Revivalism in Modern India." In: Charles Leslie (ed.), *Asian Medical Systems: A Comparative Study,* Pp. 358–367. Berkeley: University of California Press.

Leslie, Charles and Alan Young. 1992. "Introduction." In: Allan Younag and Charles Leslie (eds.), *Paths to Asian Medical Knowledge*, Pp. 1–18. Berkeley: University of California Press.

Levi-Strauss, C. 1963. *Structural Anthropology*. New York: Basic Books.

Levy, Martin. 1973. *Early Arabic Pharmacology: An Introduction Based on Ancient and Medieval Sources*. Leiden: E. J. Brill.

Lewis, Gilbert. 1993a. "Double Standards of Treatment Evaluation." In: S. Lindenbaum and M. Lock (eds.) *Knowledge, Power and Practice: The Anthropology of Medicine and Everyday Life*, Pp. 189–218. Berkeley: University of California Press.

———. 1993b. "Some Studies of Social Causes of and Cultural Response to Disease." In C. G. N. Mascie-Taylor (ed.), *The Anthropology of Disease*, Pp. 73–124. Oxford: Oxford University Press.

Lewis, Gilbert, and Stephen Frankel. 1989. "Patterns of Continuity and Change." In: Gilbert Lewis and Stephen Frankel (eds.), *A Continuing Trial of Treatment: Medical Pluralism in Papua New Guinea*, Pp. 1–33. Dordrecht, Boston, London: Kluwer Academic Publishers.

Lindenbaum, Shirley, and Margaret Lock. 1993. *Knowledge, Power and Practice: The Anthropology of Medicine and Everyday Life*. Berkeley: University of California Press.

Lock, Margaret and Vinh-Kim Nguyen. 2010. *An Anthropology of Biomedicine*. Oxford: Wiley-Blackwell, a John Wiley & Sons, Ltd., Publication.

Lock, M., and Deborah R. Gordon (eds.). 1988. *Biomedicine Examined.* Dordrecht: Kluwer Academic Publishers.

Lock, Margaret. 1993. "Cultivating the Body: Anthropologies and Epistemologies of Bodily Practice and Knowledge." *Annual Review of Anthropology* 22: 133–55.

———. 1996. "Death in Technological Time: Locating the End of Meaningful Life." Medical Anthropology Quarterly 10(4): 575–600.

———. 1996. "Displacing Suffering: The Reconstruction of Death in North America and Japan." In: Arthur Kleinman, Vena Das, and Margaret Lock, (eds.), *Social Suffering*. Berkeley: University of California Press.

———. 1997. "The Unnatural as Ideology: Contesting Brain Death in Japan." In: Pamela J. Asquith and Arne Kalland (eds.), *Japanese Images: Cultural Perspectives*. Richmond: Curzon Press.

Lock, Margaret, and Nancy Scheper-Hughes. 1990. "A Critical-Interpretive Approach in Medical Anthropology: Rituals and Routines of Discipline and Dissent." In: Thomas M. Johnson and Carolyn F. Sargent (eds), *Medical Anthropology: Contemporary Theory and Method*, Pp. 47–72. New York: Greenwood Press.

Lutfi, Safwat Hassan. 1992. *asbāb taḥrīm naql wa zirāᶜt al-'a 'ḍā' al-'ādamiyyah (the* reasons to prohibit the transplant and transfer human organs). Cairo: DN.

Lyon, M. L. and F. M. Barbalet. 1994. "Society's Body: Emotion and the 'Somatization' of Social Theory. In: Thomas J. Csordas (ed.), *Embodiment and Experience: The Existential Ground of Culture and Self*, Pp. 48–66. Cambridge: Cambridge University Press.

MacIntyre, Alasdair. 1984. *After Virtue: A Study in Moral Theory*. Notre Dame: The University of Notre Dame Press (second edition).

MacCormak, Carol P. 1981. "Health Care and the Concept of Legitimacy." *Social Science and Medicine* 15B(3): 423–428.

Maghawri, Mohammed Abdu. 1995. *Wasfaat jinniyya li al-'ilag bi al-'a'shaab al-tibbiyya* [Magical Prescriptions by Medicinal Plants]. Mansurah: maktabat al-'iman.

Mahfouz, Bey, Naguib. 1966. *Hayat Tabib*. Cairo: Dar Al-ma'arif.

———. 1935. *The History of Medical Education in Egypt*. Cairo: Government Press at *Būlāq*.

Majma'al-Lughah al-'Arabiyya [The Assembly for Arabic Language]. 1994. *Al-Mu'jam al-Wajiz* [The Brief Lexicon] Cairo: The Public Authority for Amiriyya Press.

Ma'luf, Luwis. 1997. *Al-munjid fi al-lughah wa-al-a'lam. Al-Tab'ah* 36., munaqqahah wa-mazidah. Bayrut: dar al-mashriq.

Marcus, George. 1995. "Ethnography in/of the World System: The Emergence of Multi-sited Ethnography." *Annual Review of Anthropology* 24: 95–117.

Marcus, George E., and Michael Fischer. 1986. *Anthropology as Cultural Critique: An Experimental Moment in the Human Sciences*. Chicago: The University of Chicago Press.

Martin, Emily. 1991. "The Egg and the Sperm: How Science has Constructed a Romance Based on Stereotypical Male-Female Roles." *Sings* 16: 485–501.

———. 1994. *Flexible Bodies: Tracking Immunity in American Culture from the Days of Polio to the Age of AIDS*. Boston: Beacon.

Mauss, Marcel. 1970 [1935]. "The Notion of Body Techniques." In *Sociology and Psychology*, Pp. 97–123. London: Routledge and Kegan Paul.

———. 1990 [1950]. *The Gift: The Form and Reason for Exchange in Archaic Societies*. London: Routledge.

McKinlay, J. 1985. "Introduction." In: J. McKinlay (ed.), *Issues in the Political Economy of Health Care*, Pp. 1–9. London: Tavistock.

Millar, Marcia Inhorn, and Sandra Lane. 1988. "Ethno-ophthalmology in the Egyptian Delta: An Historical Systems Approach to Ethnomedicine in the Middle East." *Social Science and Medicine* 26: 651–57.

Mishler, Elliot. 1986. *The Discourse of Medicine: Dialectics of Medical Interviews*. Norwood, N.J.: ABLEX.

Mitchell, Timothy. 1989. *Colonising Egypt*. Cairo: American University in Cairo Press.

Moosa, Ebrahim. 2005. *Ghazali and the Poetics of Imagination*. Chapel Hill and London: The University of North Carolina Press.

———. 1999. "Languages of Change in Islamic Law." *Islamic Studies* 38(3): 305–342.

Morgan, L. 1987. "Dependency Theory in the Political Economy of Health: An Anthropological Critique." *Medical Anthropology Quarterly* 1(2): 131–54.

Morgan, Lynn. 1989. "The Importance of the State in Primary Health Care Initiatives." *Medical Anthropology Quarterly* (New Series) 3(3): 227–231.

Morsy, Soheir. 1978. "Sex Roles, Power and Illness in an Egyptian Village." *American Ethnologist* 5: 137–50.

———. 1993. *Gender, Sickness, and Healing in Rural Egypt: Ethnography in Historical Context*. Boulder: Westview Press.

———. 1990. "Political Economy in Medical Anthropology." In: Thomas M. Johnson and Carolyn F. Sargent (eds.), *Medical Anthropology: Contemporary Theory and Method*, Pp. 26–46. New York: Greenwood Press.

———. 1988. "Islamic Clinics in Egypt: The Cultural Elaboration of Biomedical Hegemony." *Medical Anthropology Quarterly* 2(4): 355–67.

———. 1981. "Toward a Political Economy of Health: A Critical Note on the Medical Anthropology of the Middle East." *Social Science and Medicine* 15(B): 159–63.

———. 1980. "Body Concepts and Health Care: Illustration from an Egyptian Village." *Human Organization* 39(1): 92–96.

———. 1979. "The Missing Link in Medical Anthropology: The Political Economy of Health." *Reviews in Anthropology* 6: 349–63.

Moustafa, Tamir. 2000. "Conflict and Cooperation between the State and Religious Institutions in Contemporary Egypt." *International Journal of Middle Eastern Studies* 32: 3–22.

Mukhtar, Salem. 1993. *Al-tib al-'akhdar*: *wasfat 'ilagiyya sha'biyya* [The Green Medicine: Popular Therapeutic Prescriptions]. Cairo: maktabit ragab.

Myntti, Cynthia. 1981. "Hegemony and Healing in North Yemen." *Social Science and Medicine* 27(5): 515–20.

Nancy. 2000. "The Global Traffic in Human Organs." *Current Anthropology* 41(2): 191–210.

Nash, June. 1981. "Ethnographic Aspects of the World Capitalist System." *Annual Review of Anthropology* 10: 393–423.

Navarro, Vicente. 1986. *Crisis, Health and Medicine: A Social Critique*. New York: Tavistock Publication.

Nichter, Mark. 1980. "The Layperson's Perception of Medicine as Perspective into the Utilization of Multiple Therapy Systems in the Indian Context." *Social Science and Medicine* 14B: 225–233.

Ong, Aihwa. 1988. "The Reproduction of Possession: Spirits and the Multinational Corporation in Malaysia." *American Ethnologists* 15(1): 28–42.

Onoge, Omafome. 1975. "Capitalism and Public Health: A Neglected Topic in Medical Anthropology of Africa." In: S. R. Ingman and A. E. Thomas (eds.), *Topias and Utopias of Health*, Pp. 219–32. The Hague: Mouton.

Papagaroufali, Eleni. 1999. "Donation of Human Organs or Bodies after Death: A Cultural Phenomenology of 'Flesh' in the Greek Context." *Ethos* 27(3): 283–314.

Parkin, David. 1995. "Latticed Knowledge: Eradication and Dispersal of the Unpalatable in Islam, Medicine and Anthropological Theory." In: Richard Fardon (ed.), *Counterworks: Managing the Diversity of Knowledge*. New York: Routledge.

Population Reference Bureau. 2000. *2000 World Population Data Sheet*. Washington, D.C.: Population Reference Bureau Press

Press, Irwin. 1978. "Urban Folk Medicine." *American Anthropologist* 80: 71–84.

———. 1980. "Problems in the Definition of and Classification of Medical Systems." *Social Science and Medicine* 14B: 45–57.

Rapp, Rayna. 1993. "Accounting for Amniocentesis." In: S. Lindenbaum and M. Lock (eds.), *Knowledge, Power and Practice: The Anthropology of Medicine and Everyday Life*, Pp. 55–76. Berkeley: University of California Press.

Rebhun, L. A. 1994. "Swallowing Frogs: Anger and Illness in Northeast Brazil." *Medical Anthropology Quarterly* 8(4): 360–382.

Reymond, André. 1993. *Al-Qahira: Tarikh Hadira.* Translated into Arabic by Latif Farag. Cairo: Dar al-Fikr Liddirasat Wannashr Wattawzi'.

Rodney, W. 1974. *How Europe Underdeveloped Africa.* London: Bogle-L'Ouverture.

Rorty, Amelie. 2007. "The Vanishing Subject: The Many Faces of Subjectivity." In: Joao Biehl, Byron Good, and Arthur Kleinman (eds.), *Subjectivity: Ethnographic Investigations*, Pp. 34–51. Berkeley: University of California Press.

Rugh, Andrea. 1979. *Coping with Poverty in a Cairo Community.* Cairo Papers in Social Science Vol.1 Mon. 2.

Rugh, Andrea B. 1984. *Family in Contemporary Egypt.* Syracuse, N.Y.: Syracuse University Press.

Russel Pasha, Sir Thomas. 1949. *Egyptian Service, 1902–1946.* London: Jon Murray.

Said, Edward. 1978. *Orientalism.* New York: Random House.

Samaaha, Mohammed Riyaad. 1996. *Dalil al-mu'aalijin bi al-Quran al-karim* [Guide for Therapists by the Quran]. Cairo: al-Ahram Press.

Sandwith, F. M. 1905. *Medical Diseases of Egypt.* London: Henry Kimpton.

Scheper-Hughes, Nancy. 1990. "Three Propositions for a Critically Applied Medical Anthropology." *Social Science and Medicine*: 189–197.

Scheper-Hughes, Nancy. 2000. The Global Traffic in Human Organs. *Current Anthropology* 41(2): 191–210).

Scheper-Hughes, Nancy and Margaret Lock. 1987. "The Mindful Body: A Prolegomenon to Future Work in Medical Anthropology." *Medical Anthropology Quarterly* N.S 1(1): 6–41.

Schlecker, Markus and Eric Hirsch. 2001. "Incomplete Knowledge: Ethnography and the Crisis of Context in Studies of Media, Science and Technology." *History of the Human Sciences* 14(1): 69–87.

Schnall, Peter L. and Rochelle Kern. 1981. "Hypertension in American Society: An Introduction to Historical Materialist Epidemiology." In: Peter Conrad and Rochelle Kern (eds.), *The Sociology of Health and Illness: Critical Perspectives*, Pp. 97–121. New York: Saint Martin's Press.

Shalabi, Yasir Gaafar. 1995. *'Ilaag 'amraad al-ragul bi al'a'shaab* [Treatment of Men's Diseases by Herbs]. Cairo: al-dar al-thahabiyya lil-tibaa'a wa al-nashr wa al-tawzi'.

Sharp, Leslie. 2000. "The Commodification of the Body and Its Parts." *Annual Review of Anthropology* 29: 287–328.

Singer, Mirril. 1990. "Reinventing Medical Anthropology: Towards a Critical Realignment." *Social Science and Medicine* 30(2): 174–87.

Sonbol, Amira el Azhary. 1991. *The Creation of a Medical Profession in Egypt, 1800–1922.* Syracuse, New York: Syracuse University Press.

Strathern, Marilyn. 1992. *Reproducing the Future: Anthropology, Kinship and the New Reproductive Technologies.* Manchester: Manchester University Press.

Taussig, Michael. 1980. "Reification and the Consciousness of the Patient." *Social Science and Medicine* 14: 3–13.

Taussig, Michael. 1992. *The Nervous System.* London: Routledge, Chapman and Hall, Inc.

Tekçe, Belgin, Linda Oldham, and Fredric Shorter. 1994. *A Place to Live: Families and Child Health in a Cairo Neighbourhood.* Cairo: American University in Cairo Press.

Traweek, S. 1993. "An Introduction to Cultural and Social Studies of Science and Technology." *Culture, Medicine and Psychiatry* 17: 3.

True, William. 1990. "Epidemiology and Medical Anthropology." In: Thomas M. Johnson and Carolyn F. Sargent (eds.), *Medical Anthropology: Contemporary Theory and Method*, Pp. 298–318. New York: Greenwood Press.

Turner, Victor. 1964. "The Ndembu Doctor in Practice." In: A. Kiev (ed.), *Magic, Faith and Healing: Studies in Primitive Psychiatry Today*. New York: The Free Press.

———. 1967. *The Forest of Symbols: Aspects of Ndembu Ritual*. Ithaca and London: Cornell University Press.

Waitzkin, Howard. 1986. "Micropolotics of Medicine: Theoretical Issues." *Medical Anthropology Quarterly* 17(5): 134–36.

Wallerstein, I. 1974. *The Modern World System 1: Capitalist Agriculture and the Origins of the European World Economy in the Sixteenth Century*. New York: Academic Press.

Waterbury, John. 1978. *Egypt: Burdens of the Past, Options for the Future*. Bloomington and London: American Universities Filed Staff and University of Indiana Press.

Watson, Helen. 1992. *Women in the City of Dead*. London: Hust and Company.

Williams, Raymond. 2009. "On Structure of Feeling." In: Jennifer Harding and E. Deidre Pribram (eds.), *Emotions: A Cultural Studies Reader*, Pp. 35–49. London: London: Routledge.

Worsley, Peter. 1982. "Non-western Medical System." *Annual Review of Anthropology* 11: 315–48.

Young, Allan. 1976. "Some Implications of Medical Beliefs and Practices for Social Anthropology." *American Anthropology* 1: 257–85.

———. 1980. "The Discourse on Stress and the Reproduction of Conventional Knowledge." *Social Science and Medicine* 14B: 133–46.

———. 1981. "When Rational Men Fall Sick: An Inquiry into some Assumptions Made by Medical Anthropologists." *Culture, Medicine and Psychiatry* 5: 317–335.

———. 1982. The Anthropology of Illness and Sickness. *Annual Review of Anthropology* 11: 257–285.

———. 1993. "A Description of how Ideology Shapes Knowledge of a Mental Disorder." In: Shirely Lindenbaum and Margare Lock (eds.), *Knowledge, Power and Practice*: *The Anthropology of Medicine and Everyday Life*, Pp. 108–128. Berkeley: University of California Press.

Young, Allan and Charles Leslie (eds.). 1992. *Paths to Asian Medical Knowledge*. Berkeley: University of California Press.

Zimmerman, F. 1978. "From Classic Text to Learned Practice: Methodological Remarks on the Study of Indian Medicine." *Social Science and Medicine* 12(B): 97–103.

NEWSPAPERS

Al-Akhbar. 14.6, 1997; 5.6, 1997; 24.5, 1997; 23.5, 1997; 17.5, 1997; 10.5, 1997; 9.5, 1997; 10.2, 1996.

Al-Ahram. 19.10, 1997; 23.5, 1997; 17.5, 1997; 14.5, 1997; 7.5, 1997; 4.5, 1997; 22.4, 1997; 13.2, 1997; 31.1, 1997; 11.6, 1996; 10.6, 1996; 6.4, 1996; 24.2, 1996; 24.12, 1995; 16.12, 1995; 18.11, 1995; 28.10, 1995; 12.10, 1995; 7.10, 1995.

Al-Ahram Weekly (In English). 26.6, 1998.

Al-Dustour. 19.3, 1997; 27.11, 1996.

Al-Sha'b. 17.6, 1997; 6.4, 1997.

Al-Wafd. 9.9, 1997; 22.3, 1997; 28.1, 1996; 26.1, 1996.

Cairo Times (In English). 15–28.5, 1997.

Index

About the Author

Mohammed Tabishat, PhD, is a sociocultural anthropologist (PhD Cambridge, England 2001, MA Yarmouk University, Jordan 1992) focused on medical anthropology. Formerly, he studied medical science (BSc. Yarmouk University 1987). His work explores how health care systems constitute indexes for social structure and cultural change. Second, Tabishat is interested in psychological anthropology and the comparative studies of subjectivity as a discursive practice. Third, he has been conducting research on the notion of "tradition" and its relation to liberal arts education in the Arab region. He also developed an interest in public culture through a focus on films and the way they both represent and contribute to shaping general imagery regarding society, the individual, political struggle, and change. Key words that point to issues explored by Tabishat's work include bio-power, body politics, the political economy of heath care services, techniques of the self, sexuality, comparative forms of governance, education, and modern forms of violence and care. Tabishat conducted fieldwork in Egypt, United Arab Emerites, and Jordan. Prior to The American University in Cairo he taught anthropology at the United Arab Emerites University (Abu Dhabi) and Dickinson College (Carlisle, Pennsylvania).

www.ingramcontent.com/pod-product-compliance
Ingram Content Group UK Ltd.
Pitfield, Milton Keynes, MK11 3LW, UK
UKHW012040150926
475560UK00001B/107

9 780739 179796